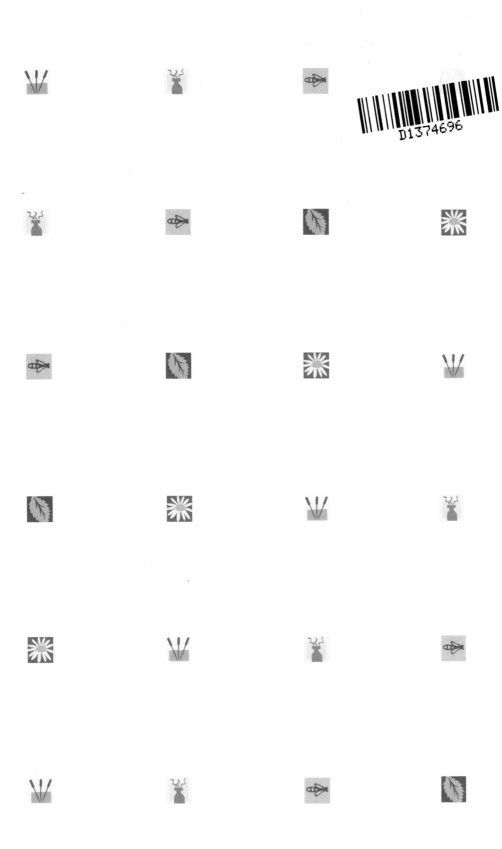

Heal Your
CAT
The Natural Way

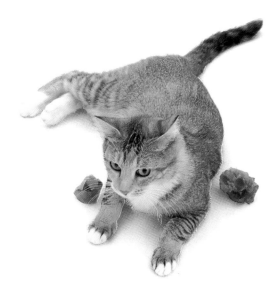

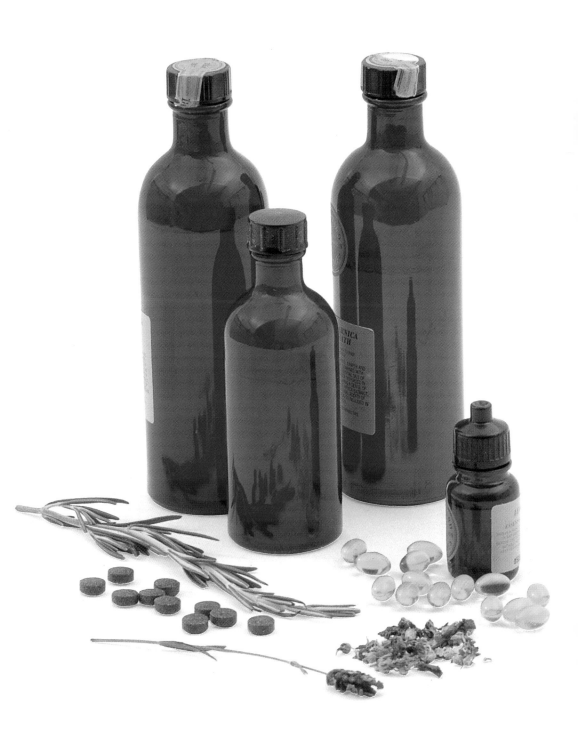

Heal Your
CAT
The Natural Way

RICHARD ALLPORT

For Maggie:

'I fear darkness, I fear night
Don't leave me empty of your light'

With thanks to Susan Lee for typing
an intelligible manuscript from my
illegible handwriting.

Senior art editor: Luise Roberts
Commissioning editor: Samantha Ward-Dutton
Project editor: Jane Royston
Copy editors: Cathy Lowne, Claire Musters
Designer: Tony Truscott
Photography: Jane Burton
Picture research: Liz Fowler
Production: Rachel Lynch

First published in Great Britain in 1997 by Mitchell Beazley,
an imprint of Reed Consumer Books Limited, Michelin House,
81 Fulham Road, London SW3 6RB and Auckland,
Melbourne, Singapore and Toronto.

ISBN 1 85732 812 4

A CIP catalogue of this book is available at the British Library.

Printed in Hong Kong

contents

introduction

As technology becomes more high-powered, as modern medicine increases in complexity, as scientific knowledge grows more all-encompassing, can there still be a place for the old remedies in the treatment of disease? With so many new drugs and a multitude of revolutionary techniques available, what need can there be for the healing power of herbs, for the holistic approach of homoeopathy, or for the ancient art of acupuncture?

There is a place and a need for these therapies – perhaps now more than ever before. The very fact that herbal treatments, homoeopathy and acupuncture, along with numerous other therapies, are currently enjoying a resurgence is a tribute to our growing awareness that natural medicines have a great deal to offer.

There are many disadvantages to the use of drugs in conventional medicine. New drugs often need to be produced because diseases have developed a resistance to their predecessors, and these are inordinately expensive and time-consuming to research, produce, test and license. Side-effects are ever-present, and new drugs often simply do not work effectively. Chronic eczema (dermatitis), disease of the immune system, chronic dysfunction of the bowel, persistent respiratory problems – each of these common problems is incurable as far as modern medicine is concerned.

It is no wonder that there has been a recent change in our attitudes to the traditional remedies. No longer are they dismissed as folklore and old wives' tales, as all over the world we are rediscovering the health-giving, healing powers of therapies that have for centuries been both safe and effective.

Many people would agree with these sentiments so far. But for cats? Can acupuncture cure an Abyssinian, or Bach flowers help a Burmese? The answer is yes. This book aims to show how natural medicines are as applicable to our feline friends as they are to us, by explaining which medicines are effective for which conditions, and by outlining in simple terms the best approaches to their use.

All you will need in order to find this book of practical help is an open mind, an interest in health – and, of course, a cat.

important note

Before starting to use this book, please remember one vital point: *Heal Your Cat The Natural Way* is NOT intended to be a substitute for seeking professional veterinary assistance for your cat whenever necessary.

Never try to diagnose and treat illness solely from the information in this book. If you are ever in any doubt about your cat's health or welfare, you must consult your vet – remember that failure to do so could put your cat's life at risk.

using this book
The first section, *natural therapies*, explores the five main therapies commonly used to treat cats – aromatherapy, homoeopathy, herbal medicine, Bach flowers and acupuncture – and then looks at various lesser-used, 'minor' therapies. With the main therapies, information is given on their origins and development, on what kind of problems should respond to them, and on how the medicines should be used to achieve the best results. A case history to illustrate the effectiveness of each therapy is included. There is also a short description of each minor therapy, with advice on its application. It is important to follow the instructions carefully, as natural remedies are not automatically completely safe – in aromatherapy, essential oils given by mouth can be toxic if given too frequently; a homoeopathic remedy in the wrong potency can aggravate symptoms.

Detailed advice is then given on how providing a suitable environment, well-chosen foods and natural supplements can help to keep a cat healthy and accelerate recovery from illness. Potential drawbacks of feeding commercial cat foods are discussed, and there is a guide to feeding a home-made diet. Many natural medicines are available in tablet form, and this section ends with clear instructions on the technique for giving tablets quickly and efficiently.

The *natural therapies* section should be used in conjunction with *common diseases and conditions* to ensure that the right therapy is administered in the correct way. In this second section, many of the common illnesses suffered by cats, and the natural remedies that can be used to relieve the symptoms, are covered. It is ordered by body systems and their ailments: for example, remedies for arthritis will be found within the musculo-skeletal system. Case studies throughout reveal the remarkable results that natural medicines can achieve.

natural

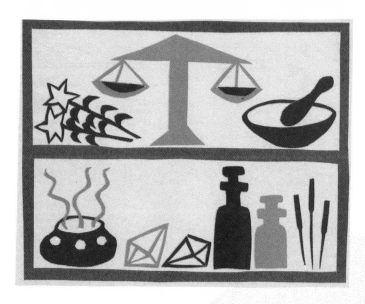

therapies

An old saying in medicine declares that there is 'a pill for every ill', and there is certainly no shortage of healing therapies for cats. The aim that is common to all the natural medicines is the restoration of balance and equilibrium to the body – a case perhaps of 'a remedy to restore order to every disorder'.

None of the therapies included in this book will have any adverse effect on conventional drugs, but you should keep your vet informed of any natural remedies that you use. Unfortunately, some conventional drugs do interfere with the efficacy of natural medicines: homoeopathic remedies and biochemical tissue salts in particular can be rendered less effective by steroids and by some hormones. However, the essential oils used in aromatherapy, herbal medicine, and flower and gem essences normally work perfectly well alongside conventional drugs.

Most natural therapies are compatible with each other, and it is quite acceptable – and often beneficial – to use more than one at a time. The only drawback here is that it can be dificult to assess which therapy is creating the greatest improvement. There are some exceptions: for example, homoeopathic remedies and biochemical tissue salts may be adversely affected by aromatic essential oils and by strong-smelling herbs (especially Garlic); similarly, it would not be wise to follow a session of osteopathy too closely with physiotherapy treatment. However, as a general rule, all the natural therapies are compatible and complementary. When given in the correct dosages, natural medicines are also very safe.

All the medicines suggested in this book should produce an obvious improvement in symptoms within the time stated: if any remedy administered in the dosage advised has no effect after a normal course of treatment, you should choose a different remedy. Of course, if your cat suffers from any acute problem that does not respond to treatment, you must consult your vet as soon as possible.

aromatherapy

Aromatherapy involves the use of essential oils derived from plants as a treatment for a range of illnesses. Although used for centuries in human ailments, aromatherapy for cats is a fairly recent development.

The essential aromatic oils are obtained by a distillation process, and the resulting product is a highly concentrated oil with – as the name implies – a strong fragrance. Each oil has its own individual properties when used as a therapeutic remedy. However, in general, essential oils are both antiseptic and detoxifying, and they help to strengthen the immune system and to regulate the metabolism. The exact mode of their action is not yet understood, but, as with all natural therapies, it seems that it is the energy within the oils that interacts with the energy in a patient to produce the healing effect.

Just some of the beneficial responses to aromatherapy include: the painkilling action of Lavender and Marjoram; the anti-arthritic effect of Juniper, Pine and Sandalwood; improvement in digestive problems following the use of Caraway and Coriander; and the relief of respiratory symptoms with Eucalyptus and Thyme.

treatment

There are three main ways to administer essential oils: by mouth (oral administration), by massage and by using a diffuser.

oral administration

Oils can be given by mouth, but this method should only be used under the strict supervision of an expert in aromatherapy. This is because the essential oils are so highly concentrated that even small quantities can have a toxic effect.

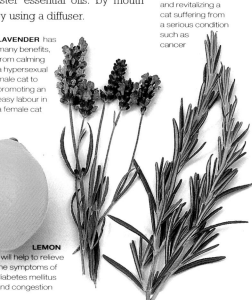

ROSEMARY is a widely used herb that is especially useful in relieving arthritic stiffness and revitalizing a cat suffering from a serious condition such as cancer

LAVENDER has many benefits, from calming a hypersexual male cat to promoting an easy labour in a female cat

LEMON will help to relieve the symptoms of diabetes mellitus and congestion

Aromatherapy oils are obtained from a wide range of plants, fruits and herbs. Given via massage or diffusion, they often produce good results in cases that have not responded to treatment with conventional drugs.

massage

This method is most commonly used. One drop of the appropriate oil is added to 2.5 ml (½ tsp) of an inert 'carrier' oil such as Wheatgerm, Sweet-almond or Sunflower. The role of a carrier is to dilute the essential oil, allowing it to be absorbed easily through the cat's skin. A few drops of the diluted mixture are massaged into a hairless – or the least hairy – area of skin (usually the 'armpit' area, the groin, or an inner thigh). Three to four minutes of gentle massage will allow sufficient oil to be absorbed into the skin. The majority of aromatherapists will suggest twice-daily massage for five days as a typical regime. Neat essential oils must never be applied to the skin, as they can cause soreness.

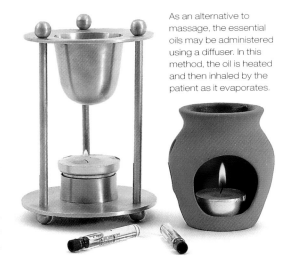

As an alternative to massage, the essential oils may be administered using a diffuser. In this method, the oil is heated and then inhaled by the patient as it evaporates.

diffusion

In this technique a diffuser evaporates the oil, which is then inhaled by the patient. The diffuser should be left in operation with the cat in the same room for 30 minutes so that sufficient oil is absorbed. This should be repeated twice daily for five days. Diffusers are inexpensive to buy and come with simple setting-up instructions.

suitability

Aromatherapy has a rapid action – a few days' treatment is normally all that is required – and the fragrant remedies are very pleasant to use. They are also readily available: health-food stores, pharmacies and even beauty-product outlets stock or can obtain essential oils.

The disadvantages involve administering the oils to a cat. As has been discussed, oral dosing is not normally advisable, while massage can sometimes be a problem: most cats do seem to appreciate a gentle massage for a few minutes each day, but some become bored and can be difficult to keep still. Diffusers can also be messy and are time-consuming to use. One further drawback of aromatherapy is the cost: essential oils are expensive, and have only a limited shelf-life.

aromatherapy case study

Blackie was – as you would expect – a black cat, very big and bold, and a terror to the local cat population. If he had been human he would doubtless have been categorized as the neighbourhood troublemaker: out roaming the streets at all hours of the night, tormenting the local youngsters and even becoming involved in petty theft (he once brought home half a joint of roast lamb, whose source was never ascertained).

However, although a physically strong cat, Blackie suffered from chronic nasal congestion. He had been afflicted by feline upper-respiratory-tract disease – a condition commonly known as cat 'flu (see page 118) – as a kitten, and, despite making a good recovery, was left with a persistently blocked nose. No amount of antibiotics or decongestants could solve the problem.

When I suggested a course of aromatherapy, Blackie's owner was doubtful that carrying out the treatment would be possible. Blackie hated being indoors, and she felt that staying in a room with a diffuser for more than a few minutes would be purgatory for him. For this reason, she reluctantly agreed to try massage. One drop each of Eucalyptus and Thyme was added to 2.5 ml (½ tsp) of Sunflower oil, and this mixture was massaged into Blackie's flank and abdomen for three minutes twice daily.

I saw Blackie again two weeks later and heard, to my surprise, that he had been a perfect patient during treatment. His owner had brought some oil with her, and demonstrated the way in which Blackie lay absolutely still while she gently massaged the oil into his skin. If only the neighbourhood cats could have seen their tormentor lying there, purring loudly as his owner massaged him into a state of ecstasy, his street credibility would have disappeared instantly. Even more surprisingly, Blackie's congestion, as well as the nasal discharge, had – even after this short period of treatment – already begun to diminish noticeably.

I recommended that, from this point onwards, Blackie should be massaged twice a week. When I next saw him, eight weeks later, he seemed to be cured: his nostrils were clean, and there was no snuffling or congestion. No further treatment was required, but, as he evidently enjoyed the massage so much, his owner decided to continue with it once a week regardless.

homoeopathy

In the late 18th century doctors were probably killing as many patients as they cured, bloodletting was still practised, and many 'medicines' were actually poisons. However, a German doctor called Samuel Hahnemann developed a system of medicine – based on lengthy observation and rigorous experimentation – that he called homoeopathy. Today, it is an irony that homoeopathy is often derided as unscientific by some members of the medical establishment, when in fact it was founded purely on scientific principles in an age of quackery in medicine.

Hahnemann found that a substance of mineral, plant or animal origin that causes adverse symptoms in an individual could cure those same symptoms when given in a minute, 'energized' homoeopathic dose. So, for instance, Arsenic would cause a bout of severe gastro-enteritis if swallowed, yet homoeopathic Arsenic would actually cure the symptoms of the condition.

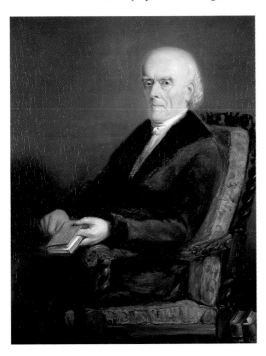

The German physician Dr Samuel Hahnemann (1755–1843), the founder of homoeopathy.

Homoeopathic remedies are produced by diluting the original substance in several stages, and by shaking, or 'succussing', the solution at each dilution to add energy to the product. This system of increasingly diluting but also energizing the starting material results in remedies that are so dilute as to be completely safe and free from side-effects, yet are powerful enough to act as strong healing agents.

Remedies are made from minerals such as Lead, Arsenic and Phosphorus; from plants such as Belladonna, Aconite and Arnica; and from animal products ranging from the honeybee (Apis mellifica, commonly known as Apis mel.) to the venom of poisonous snakes (for instance, Lachesis). There are over 3000 different homoeopathic remedies in use, all working on Hahnemann's principle that 'like cures like' – a remedy given in a small dose will cure the symptoms caused by the material substance.

Hahnemann also found that homoeopathic remedies corresponded to the mental and emotional states of a patient. For example, an individual who would benefit from homoeopathic arsenic tended to be anxious and restless, to seek warmth, to drink small amounts of fluids frequently, and to dislike cold, wet weather. On the other hand, a lazy, overweight, relaxed character who lived to eat, drink and sleep would be a candidate for homoeopathic Calcarea carbonica (Calc. carb.).

This idea of a homoeopathic 'constitution' – that is, the concept that each individual person (or animal) is a particular physical, mental and emotional type and will correspond to a particular homoeopathic remedy – is especially useful when dealing with chronic and deepseated disease. Homoeopathy can be used to treat almost all diseases found in cats, but it is especially effective for chronic conditions such as skin disorders, arthritis and longstanding respiratory problems.

Homoeopathic remedies are commonly known by abbreviations of their Latin names, and have been listed as such in the *common diseases and conditions* section of this book. The full names of the remedies may be found on page 126.

treatment

Homoeopathic remedies are available as tablets, powders, granules (pillules), liquids and ointments. Ointments can be applied directly to the affected area (they should be applied two to three times daily), but tablets are the most widely available form of homoeopathic remedies. The dosage rates quoted in this book are applicable to this form of medication and are as follows:

For acute conditions, give one tablet every 15 minutes for three hours, then one tablet hourly for the rest of the day. After this, give one tablet three times daily for three further days, or until all symptoms have disappeared.

For chronic conditions, give one tablet three times daily for one week, followed by one tablet twice daily for three weeks.

If other forms of remedy are used, the equivalent doses are:
one tablet = one powder = 12 granules = three drops of liquid.

Remedies are also produced in different potencies. The commonly available potency is known as 6c, and this will be marked on the tablet container. The correct remedy for a condition will be effective in any potency, but the higher the potency (the larger the number before the 'c') the greater the healing action will be. However, if too high a potency is given the symptoms may temporarily become aggravated, so you should use 6c potencies only (unless advised otherwise by a vet with expertise in homoeopathy).

Homoeopathic remedies should be given by mouth, if possible. This should be done away from food and without touching the tablets, as their effectiveness can be reduced by certain chemicals in foodstuffs and even by traces of chemicals on fingers. (Herbs with powerful aromas – such as Garlic – may also reduce the potency of homoeopathic remedies, and should not be given at the same time.) It is usually possible to shake a tablet from the container into the cap, then to drop it from the cap into the cat's mouth; alternatively, a special syringe is available for giving tablets (see page 49).

Some manufacturers make soft tablets that dissolve in the mouth within a few seconds; however, most tablets on the market are hard and take a little longer to be absorbed. As homoeopathic tablets are absorbed better through the lining of the mouth, rather than through the stomach after being swallowed, it may be preferable to crush a hard tablet into a powder first, in a folded sheet of clean paper. The paper can then be 'funnelled' to tip the powder into the cat's mouth.

A tablet can be given with a little butter to help it to slip down the throat more easily. However, it should not be mixed with a large quantity of food, as the effectiveness of absorption may be reduced; nor should it be given within 30 minutes either side of a meal.

On many tablet containers you will see instructions such as 'two tablets for an adult, one for a child'. In fact, as a homoeopathic preparation is giving the body an energy input rather than a physical substance, the dose is the same for all animals (including humans) of any size. There is not twice the effect when giving two tablets, and a single tablet is all that is ever necessary at any one time. The only reason that manufacturers put this instruction on the label is because they believe that we expect an adult to take a larger dose than a child!

storing homoeopathic remedies

Store homoeopathic remedies away from strong smells, bright light and excessive heat or cold. Magnetic fields from electrical equipment can also render the medicines less effective. Although this makes homoeopathic products sound very fragile, if stored correctly they will remain active for years.

homoeopathy case study

Marron was an unusual-looking cat who, when young, had had a rich, chestnut-coloured coat. When I saw him he had a moth-eaten, muddy-brown appearance. His skin was badly infected, sore and mainly bald. He was four years old, and from the age of six months the condition of his skin had been steadily deteriorating. Many conventional drugs had been used over the years, but to no avail.

I saw Marron as one of my first referral cases in homoeopathy and, looking at the extent of the problem, at its longevity and at its resistance to treatment, my heart sank. I took a detailed case history, and felt no wiser; my brain raced through possible homoeopathic remedies, but no particular one appeared to fit all the symptoms. However, something that the owner had said – that Marron had never been well since being neutered – reminded me of something a homoeopathy lecturer had emphasized time and again: 'Always look out for the "never-well-since" syndrome.' In homoeopathy, it is vital to examine events surrounding the onset of disease. If a patient has not been fully well since a particular incident, the homoeopath must treat what happened then, even if it occurred months earlier.

Apparently Marron had been a sweet, loving, healthy kitten, with shining fur. After being neutered, he had become a spiteful, bad-tempered cat, and soon developed a skin condition that rapidly worsened – and never improved. Marron's owner even said: 'He always seemed resentful of us afterwards.' I felt that Marron had never recovered from the distress of being sent to a strange place and undergoing a frightening experience, and that his resentment had caused both the change in his behaviour and his skin condition.

The homoeopathic remedy Staphisagria (from the stavesacre plant) is used precisely where there are feelings of resentment, and where physical disease seems to start because of it. I prescribed a 10-day course for Marron, and awaited developments.

This single course produced a remarkable change. Within a few days the skin was improving, by the end of the course new fur was growing, and four weeks later Marron's skin and coat were almost back to normal. His personality had also changed dramatically – he became the loving cat he had been before his operation. No further treatment was necessary: one course was enough to release the anger and resentment, and to allow a natural healing to occur.

herbal medicine

Herbal medicine, or phytotherapy as it is more correctly known, is probably the oldest system of natural medicine used by human beings. Nothing could be more natural than harnessing the healing powers of the herbs and flowers around us to cure our diseases and those of our pets; indeed, animals in the wild have an uncanny ability to seek out and eat plants that will help them when they are ill or injured.

Modern drugs may be isolated extracts of herbs, or – more commonly – are synthetic derivatives of these substances. Aspirin (obtained from the bark of the willow tree) and Digitalis (from the foxglove) are two drugs with herbal origins that are still in widespread use today. However, isolated extracts and synthetic compounds are more likely to cause side-effects, and have less overall healing power

Herbal medicine aims not only to treat symptoms, but to restore normal bodily functions so that natural healing can occur. Over 2000 medicinal plants are used today, many of which have been revered for their healing properties since ancient times.

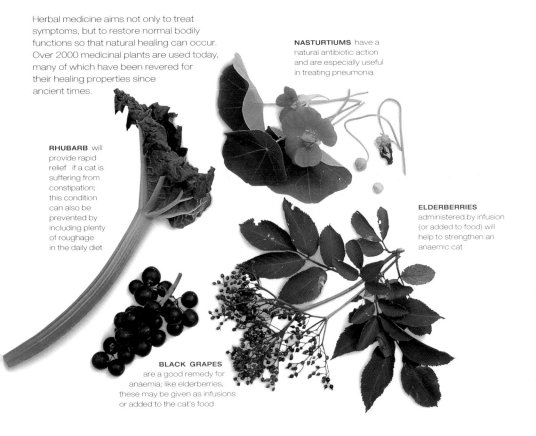

NASTURTIUMS have a natural antibiotic action and are especially useful in treating pneumonia

RHUBARB will provide rapid relief if a cat is suffering from constipation; this condition can also be prevented by including plenty of roughage in the daily diet

ELDERBERRIES administered by infusion (or added to food) will help to strengthen an anaemic cat

BLACK GRAPES are a good remedy for anaemia; like elderberries, these may be given as infusions or added to the cat's food

than the herbs themselves. Herbal medicines are more gentle and safe, yet are no less effective than their conventional counterparts.

treatment

Herbal remedies may be obtained from herbalist shops, or can be prepared at home from wild plants such as Nettles and Dandelions.

proprietary herbal remedies

Many are available for cats, usually in tablet form. This makes dosing easier, as tablets are often more acceptable to cats than infusions. Tinctures and lotions are also available, and are easy to administer. If given by mouth, a tincture should be undiluted, but a tincture used for the eyes should be diluted by adding three drops to 10 ml (2 tsps) of sterile water. For all products, follow the instructions on the packaging, and take care not to overdose.

infusions

Some herbs are not yet available as tablets, tinctures or lotions. The standard way to administer a herb of this type is by infusion.

Take 1 tsp of the dried herb, and pour on a cup of boiling water. Leave this to stand for approximately 20 minutes. Strain the mixture, allow to cool, and the infusion is ready.

An infusion will remain active for several days if kept cool, but many herbalists recommend making a fresh mixture every two days. Give 10 ml (2 tsps) twice daily with food for one week for an acute condition; for a chronic condition, give the same dose but continue for eight weeks.

decoctions

Herbs that consist of roots, bark or other hard tissue should be used to make up what is known as a decoction. To do this,

Herbal infusions and decoctions are simple to make, and will remain useable for several days if kept stored in cool and dry conditions.

simply add the chosen herb to boiling water, at the rate of 15 ml (3 tsps) per 300 ml (½ pt) of water. Keep this mixture at boiling point for 20 minutes, then strain and allow to cool. Administer as for an infusion.

If you gather your own herbs, make sure they have not been treated with pesticides. Ideally, use freshly picked herbs on the same day, or air-dry them in a well-ventilated room (keep the herbs well-separated, not bunched together). Once dried, keep them in airtight containers and use within 12 months.

suitability

Herbal remedies seem particularly effective for chronic problems. For instance, Skullcap combined with Valerian is helpful for persistent hyperactive behaviour, and Yarrow and Burdock help to alleviate arthritis. If herbal medicines are given correctly, their gentle action and long history of effectiveness make them an ideal treatment for many conditions. All the herbs in the *common diseases and conditions* section of this book can be used safely in the dosages specified here.

However, some of the lesser-used herbs can be difficult to obtain, and preparing and giving infusions or decoctions can be time-consuming. A cat's response to herbal medicine can also be slow, and it may take up to two weeks before you see any obvious improvement in the symptoms. You may then need to continue with the treatment for several months for maximum benefit.

Most importantly, there is a risk of giving too little or too much: overdosing with some remedies can be fatal. Always use herbal remedies specifically made for cats, and give them according to the package directions or on the advice of a vet familiar with herbal medicine.

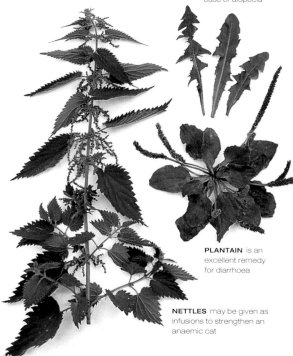

DANDELION will help to relieve the symptoms of a range of diseases, including arthritis, liver disease and recurrent cystitis; it may also promote hair regrowth in a case of alopecia

PLANTAIN is an excellent remedy for diarrhoea

NETTLES may be given as infusions to strengthen an anaemic cat

Many herbs are common in our countryside, but rare species must only be obtained from a herbalist.

herbal-medicine case study

Germaine was a Siamese cat afflicted by the distressing physical problem of recurrent diarrhoea. After an initial bout of diarrhoea as a kitten, which had been cleared up with antibiotics, she began to experience repeated spells of the same problem. Every few weeks, her long-suffering owners recognized the frequent trips to the litter tray, the straining, and the unpleasant odour of the diarrhoea.

Over months and years, every treatment known to vets had been tried, and every investigation performed, to no effect. No cause for the diarrhoea had ever been found and, although antibiotics and steroids were effective in suppressing the symptoms, nothing kept the problem at bay for long.

When Germaine was referred to me she had just started another bout of diarrhoea, and I prescribed two herbal remedies: Garlic and Slippery elm. Garlic is known as 'nature's disinfectant', and acts in the intestines by killing bacteria that can cause disease and infection, allowing a restoration of the normal, beneficial bacterial population. Slippery elm is the powdered bark from the tree of that name, and is a soothing herbal medicine. It reduces bowel inflammation and irritation, and 'tones' the intestinal lining to improve bowel function.

Germaine started with a course of Slippery elm. This was administered in tablet form, as a 10-day course of 400 mg per day (slippery elm is also available as a loose powder). Cats can be difficult to medicate, but Germaine tolerated her daily tablets well. By the end of the course the diarrhoea had ceased, and Germaine was producing what her delighted owners described as the 'best-quality' faeces for many months.

I then put Germaine on Garlic. At first, ⅓ clove of raw Garlic, chopped finely, was added to her food. This caused an instant hunger strike, so we changed to Garlic-oil capsules, with one 2 mg capsule given twice daily. After 10 days of Garlic, I advised giving 5 ml (1 tsp) of live yoghurt twice daily: this contains lactobacillus bacteria, which help to repopulate the intestines with a range of beneficial bacteria once the harmful ones have been destroyed.

Germaine never looked back. Although still prone to the odd bout of diarrhoea, this now occurs once or twice a year, not once or twice a month. During an episode the same herbal treatment quickly provides relief, and controls the problem for a long period.

Bach flowers

The Bach flower essences are named after Dr Edward Bach, a highly respected bacteriologist and homoeopath who worked for many years at the Royal London Homoeopathic Hospital. He then turned his attention to the healing powers of flowers, plants and trees, and – first in Wales and later in Oxfordshire – immersed himself in studying their potential for resolving mental and emotional problems. Dr Bach felt that physical illness and mental states are closely linked and that, by stabilizing and balancing mental or spiritual problems, physical disease would be cured as a follow-on process.

Dr Bach developed a process of 'energizing' the healing potential of the energy within flowers. He found that the action of sunlight on the petals (or other parts) of chosen plants that were floated in water would

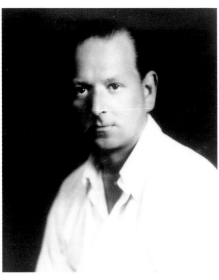

transfer the healing energy from the plant into the water. He then added a few drops of this energized water to brandy, which acted as a preservative, and the resulting mixture was Bach flower essence.

Over the following years, Dr Bach created 38 flower essences, each of which has a specific effect on mental, emotional or behavioural problems. For instance, Aspen produces a remedy beneficial for anxiety, vague fears and apprehensions; Impatiens is used to treat feelings of irritability, impatience and over-reaction; Mimulus is helpful for specific fears such as fear of noise or of the dark, as well as for general shyness and timidity; and Vine

Dr Edward Bach developed his range of flower essences to treat mental, emotional and behavioural problems, which he considered to be linked to physical disease.

is the source of a remedy that can overcome strong feelings of dominance and a need for power. If a physical illness seems to be linked with a mental or emotional problem, the therapy will almost certainly relieve the symptoms of the physical disease as well.

In addition to the 38 single remedies, a further Bach flower product was developed from a mixture of five of the original essences, and its components have a remarkable effect in cases of shock, collapse and trauma. The combination is known as Rescue Remedy, and is probably the best-known of the Bach flower range. It is an ideal component of a first-aid kit, and can be a life-saver.

treatment

Depending on the ailment, it is quite common when using Bach flower essences to give more than one remedy at a time.

Bach flowers

The essences can be administered directly by mouth (see opposite): to avoid contamination, take care to ensure that the dosing pipette does not touch the cat's mouth. Alternatively, you can add the essences to drinking water or to a small amount of food. When taken by humans, the remedy is normally diluted, and then four drops given four times daily. Cats seem to respond better to the 'neat' essence, given as one drop twice daily: it is difficult to persuade a cat to take any mixture four times a day! Continue the treatment for at least four weeks to achieve the full effect; it can be given for longer periods if symptoms recur.

Rescue Remedy

This should be used at times of accident and trauma. In this case, give one drop every five minutes for one hour, or until a change to other treatment is made.

tablets

Bach flowers are also available in the form of proprietary tablets; refer to the instructions on the container for dosage. (For the technique of giving tablets, see page 49.)

suitability

Bach flower remedies are readily available (most health-food stores stock or can obtain them), and the range is small and straightforward. It is generally easier to pick one of 38 Bach flowers than one of over 3000 homoeopathic remedies, or over 2000 medicinal plants used in herbal medicine! They are also simple to administer (drops are usually easier than tablets where cats are concerned).

Disadvantages are that this therapy is restricted to problems associated with behaviour or the emotions; it is also vitally important to understand a cat's state of mind to use Bach flowers effectively. Treatment is fairly long-term (there are no side-effects, so this is perfectly safe): dosage for four to eight weeks is necessary in most cases to obtain the full effect. When the desired result has been achieved, therapy can often be discontinued, but in some cases it may be required indefinitely to maintain the improvement.

giving Bach flower essence

I Draw the essence into the dropper. Hold the cat's head and gently tilt it back. Use the thumb of the other hand to draw down the lower jaw, and gently squeeze with the fingers of the first hand to keep the jaws apart.

2 Pick up the dropper, and hold it over the cat's mouth (do not touch the mouth, to avoid contamination of the dropper), using a finger to keep the jaws open. Administer the liquid, then release the cat's head.

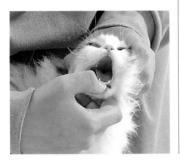
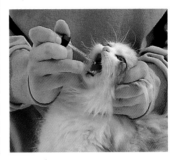

Bach flowers case study

Brandy was a thin, nervous cat, brought to see me by an owner who also had two other cats. Whisky and Soda had been in residence for years; Brandy had arrived a few weeks earlier. Whisky and Soda resented the newcomer bitterly, attacked him on sight – and continued to do so. A state of armed neutrality had been reached only by keeping the warring parties separated: Brandy was confined to one room, to which Whisky and Soda were not allowed access. This state of affairs was highly unsatisfactory, so my help was sought.

As the problems involved were behavioural, Bach flowers seemed a logical choice. For Whisky and Soda I suggested the remedies of Vine (for dominance), Holly (for jealousy and hatred) and Willow (for resentment). Brandy was given Mimulus (for specific fears), Walnut (for difficulties in adjusting to transitions in life) and Rock rose (for terror and panic). All three cats were given one drop of each remedy twice daily.

Six weeks later, I received a package in the post, containing two items. One was a photograph of Brandy, Whisky and Soda curled up together, fast asleep; the other was a small bottle of brandy. I think the treatment had worked.

acupuncture

Acupuncture is the ancient Chinese art of inserting needles at selected points in the body. It has a venerable history, with treatment recorded as many as 3000 years ago.

The traditional Chinese belief is that energy flows through the body along channels, or meridians, and that disease is caused by an imbalance or blockage in this energy flow. By inserting fine needles at specific points along the meridians, the energy flow can be stimulated, sedated or balanced, and, in this way, healing will begin to occur.

This philosophy is the starting point for the treatment of a whole range of diseases. Acupuncture therapy can be used for almost any condition, but is especially helpful for problems in the musculo-skeletal system (such as arthritis, back pain, and ligament injuries), and in the nervous system (such as trapped nerves and paralysis).

Acupuncture is probably most widely known for its effectiveness in relieving pain, but it is much more than simply an unusual form of painkiller. It can aid the healing of damaged tissue, help to regenerate nerves and stimulate the immune system – these are just some of the many ways in which this therapy can be a powerful agent for treating illness in cats.

Acupuncture needles are sterile and are used once only. The treatment involves minimal discomfort if the patient can be persuaded to remain still.

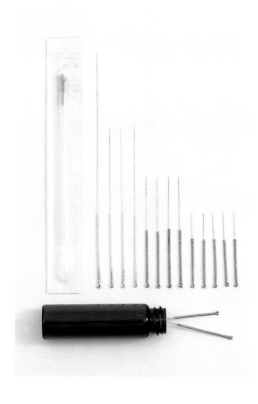

treatment

Acupuncture therapy must only be carried out on a cat by a vet who has been fully trained in the technique. Never attempt to use acupuncture needles yourself. This type of therapy generally involves one session per week initially. Once improvement has occurred, sessions may graduate to four-weekly – or even longer – intervals if continuing treatment is necessary. In most cases a response to treatment will be seen within three sessions; if no improvement is noticeable after this time, it is unlikely that further acupuncture will be of benefit.

Treatment with acupuncture will vary from, for instance, a cat with a sprained shoulder requiring six needles inserted once a week for three or four weeks – resulting in a lasting cure – to an old cat with chronic spinal arthritis, requiring 12 needles inserted once a week for six weeks, then once a month for six months, followed by a 'booster' session every two or three months for life. A cure is not expected for this kind of problem, but the acupuncture will certainly help to control the pain and stiffness.

Cats are rather variable in their acceptance of acupuncture needling. Those who are normally well-behaved when visiting the vet, or who can be held still without becoming restless, tolerate the procedure surprisingly well. However, cats who tend to resent being handled for any length of time, or who are very wriggly, can be less suitable for acupuncture therapy.

Once the needles are in place, they are quite painless provided that the patient remains still: in fact, many cats become relaxed and tranquil during sessions. However, cats who try to move about may experience some discomfort. When I was training in acupuncture, one of my lecturers told me about such a problem. He had just inserted several needles in a feline patient, when the cat in question began to twitch his skin. This caused the needles to move, which was evidently quite uncomfortable as the cat suddenly sprang on to the vet's head and ran down his back! Luckily, such events are rare, and with careful handling most cats can be successfully treated.

With the majority of cats, simple needling is perfectly sufficient. However, one or more of the following three alternative forms of acupuncture may be used in those few cases where needles on their own are not producing the desired response.

electro-acupuncture

With this technique, electrodes are attached to the needles and a small electric current passes through the needles into the acupuncture point. This is said to amplify the healing effect.

moxibustion

In this form of acupuncture, the dried Chinese herb, Moxa, is burned, and the resulting heat applied either directly to the needle, or to the skin over the acupuncture point. Using heat in this way is thought to enhance the healing effect; the Chinese also believe that Moxa itself is a herb with healing properties.

laser treatment

A more modern form of acupuncture involves focusing a laser beam on the acupuncture point. This has the advantage of being painless, but the disadvantage of requiring the use of expensive equipment.

suitability

Acupuncture can be used extremely successfully to treat a host of feline problems, from sinusitis to skin disease. The benefits of this therapy include its rapid painkilling effect, and the fact that between sessions no tablets or other treatments are required to maintain that effect. As the needles are sterile and used only once, there is no health risk. The only possible 'side-effect' is that a few cats experience a temporary aggravation of symptoms. This 'getting worse before getting better' is common to many of the natural therapies. It is not a true side-effect as compared with conventional drugs, but is simply a natural reaction of the body as it begins to throw off the disease.

Disadvantages are few: mainly that some cats are anxious when needles are inserted, and that the nearest vet practising acupuncture may be some distance away, making travel to regular sessions difficult.

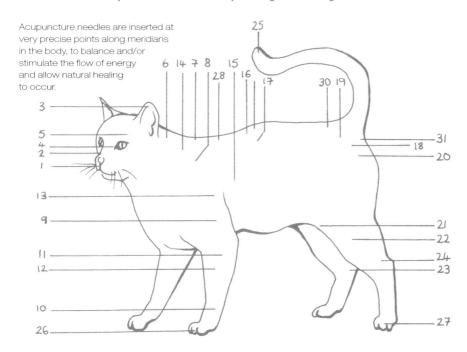

Acupuncture needles are inserted at very precise points along meridians in the body, to balance and/or stimulate the flow of energy and allow natural healing to occur.

acupuncture case study

Spliffy was a long-haired black-and-white cat of uncertain pedigree: in other words, what many people would call a stray moggy. He had been rescued after a road-traffic accident by a passing veterinary nurse, and so was lucky enough to receive rapid and expert attention to his damaged body.

Unfortunately, one of Spliffy's many injuries was a crushed spine. Although he recovered from all his other injuries, the spinal damage left him with a weak bladder and paralysed hindlegs. This meant that Spliffy, now in the permanent care of the veterinary nurse, had to have his bladder emptied for him by a process of manual squeezing – an undignified procedure that he obviously hated.

Spliffy's new owner was very interested in acupuncture therapy, and we decided to see whether needling would be beneficial. Treatment began, using six needles per session. Points needled included Weizhong (a point for back pain and spinal damage) and Qihai (a point that helps to restore normal bladder function). There are hundreds of different acupuncture points, not all of which have individual names, but certain points tend to be used more frequently than others and are distinguished in this way. Thankfully, unlike some feline patients, Spliffy was the model of patience when the needles were put in position.

We started with three sessions, at weekly intervals, with the needles left in place for 10 minutes on each occasion. Within those first three sessions, an improvement was visible. Spliffy had more energy, began to demonstrate increased strength in his hindlegs, and started to regain a little bladder control. Sessions continued at weekly intervals for another three weeks, were changed to two-week intervals for a further six weeks, and were then reduced to four-week intervals for six months.

During this period Spliffy showed a gradual and sustained improvement. His hindlegs became strong enough for him to jump out of his basket to greet me in the consulting room – when I first saw him, he had had to be lifted out. He had also regained reasonable bladder control, and so was saved the indignity of needing to have it emptied for him. Although he still had a tendency to leave small damp patches behind him from time to time, life was much better and easier for all concerned.

minor therapies
In addition to the main therapies described so far, there is a wide range of other natural therapies that may be used in the treatment of disease in cats. Most of these are included in the following list, and are therapies that I have used on feline patients, with varying degrees of success. There are a few other treatments, not described here: these have been omitted either because I have no personal experience of their use, or have not sufficient evidence that cats would respond to them.

biochemical tissue salts

Biochemical tissue salts were the discovery of a German doctor called William Schuessler. His theory was that, for body tissue to function in the best way, the cells must have a healthy balance of the 12 mineral salts that form a large part of the cells' composition. The minerals used are 'energized' as in homoeopathy, but only to a low potency; the energized mineral remedy (or a combination of several remedies) is then used as a treatment for a wide variety of conditions. Schuessler, by trial and experiment, discovered which tissue salts would be effective for which diseases.

Biochemical tissue therapy is by nature similar to homoeopathy, and can be used to treat a range of diseases. In general, tissue salts are very effective in the treatment of physical disease, although, as there are only 12 remedies in the range compared with the thousands of homoeopathic remedies, the effects are often less specific.

The 12 tissue salts are commonly known by abbreviations of their Latin names, and have been listed as such in the *common diseases and conditions* section of this book. The salts are as follows: Calcarea fluorica (Calc. fluor.), Calcarea phosphorica (Calc. phos.), Calcarea sulphurica (Calc. sulph.), Ferrum phosphoricum (Ferr. phos.), Kali muriaticum (Kali mur.), Kali phosphoricum (Kali phos.), Kali sulphuricum (Kali sulph.), Magnesia phosphorica (Mag. phos.), Natrum muriaticum (Nat. mur.), Natrum phosphoricum (Nat. phos.), Natrum sulphuricum (Nat. sulph.) and Silica (not abbreviated).

treatment

As biochemical tissue salts are produced in a similar way to homoeopathic remedies, and are available in the form of proprietary tablets, the instructions for dosage are exactly the same as for homoeopathic preparations (see pages 14–15; see also page 49 for how to administer tablets).

Chinese medicine

Traditional oriental medicine has three main strands: herbal medicine (see pages 17–20), acupuncture (see pages 24–7) and food cures. The approach is a holistic one, so a practitioner may well use a combination of all three therapies.

The Chinese version of herbal medicine is somewhat different from the Western equivalent. Chinese phytotherapy involves the use of many different herbs, fungi and even shells, simmered for a long period with water until a concentrated liquid remains.

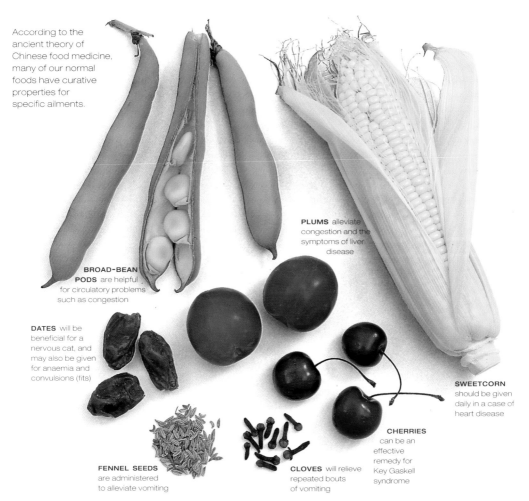

According to the ancient theory of Chinese food medicine, many of our normal foods have curative properties for specific ailments.

PLUMS alleviate congestion and the symptoms of liver disease

BROAD-BEAN PODS are helpful for circulatory problems such as congestion

DATES will be beneficial for a nervous cat, and may also be given for anaemia and convulsions (fits)

SWEETCORN should be given daily in a case of heart disease

CHERRIES can be an effective remedy for Key Gaskell syndrome

FENNEL SEEDS are administered to alleviate vomiting

CLOVES will relieve repeated bouts of vomiting

In the dietary field, Chinese medicine views foods as treatments for disease. In general terms, pungent foods (such as ginger and onion) are warming and promote energy circulation. Sweet foods (such as honey and sugar) neutralize the toxic effects of other foods, and slow down acute symptom development. Sour foods (such as lemons and plums) are helpful for diarrhoea. Bitter foods (such as hops and radishes) reduce fever, but have a laxative effect. Salty foods (such as kelp and seaweed) soften hardened tissue, thus relieving muscle spasm and alleviating enlarged lymph glands.

treatment

Cats may not be suitable patients for a total application of Chinese medicine, as the concentrated liquid produced in phytotherapy is foul-tasting, and I have yet to meet a cat who would accept it. However, the same principles do apply as for humans, and a modified treatment using acupuncture, Western herbal medicine and a sprinkling of Chinese food cures where applicable is certainly an option. (For acupuncture methods, refer to pages 24–7; Chinese food cures are included where applicable in the *common diseases and conditions* section, along with their dosages and methods of administration.)

flower therapies

As well as Bach flower remedies (see pages 21–3), other lesser known but very effective essences are available. For instance, the Bailey flower essences are of great value, as are the Australian and Alaskan essences. There is even a Hawaiian aloha flower-essence range!

All these essences act primarily at the level of the mental state of the patient, and so have a particular relevance for behavioural problems, or for cats experiencing grief following the loss of a friend (feline or human), or distress or unhappiness in a boarding cattery.

treatment

Dosage rates for all these flower essences are as for Bach flower remedies (see pages 22–3).

T-touch massage

This is a type of massage developed by Linda Tellington-Jones, an American animal behaviourist, and is derived from the human massage and movement technique of Moshe Feldenkrais. T-touch is a system of gentle, repeated massaging movements that are said to generate specific brainwave patterns in the patient. The massage is beneficial for cats suffering from anxieties, and especially for those recovering from injuries or surgery. It helps to calm a cat so that the healing is both mental and physical.

treatment

The basic T-touch massage is a series of small, circular massage movements, as if pushing the fingers around a clockface, starting at six and pushing the skin slowly clockwise all the way round, past six again and finishing at eight. These massage circles are performed randomly all over the body and continued for about 15 minutes. This procedure is repeated two or three times per day.

Massage sessions of 15 minutes should be given three times a day for a week in acute conditions, and for four weeks in chronic disorders.

reflexology

This is a way of treating disease in body organs by applying pressure to particular points. Although its use was known in India and China 5000 years ago, the American doctor, W T Fitzgerald, founded modern reflexology. He discovered that by applying pressure to his (human) patients' hands he could relieve pain. This technique was developed by Eunice Ingham into the better-known foot reflexology.

Although the anatomy of a cat's foot is somewhat different from our own, the reflexology principles hold good.

treatment

The theory that certain areas of the feet and hands correspond to certain organs and glands is related to the theory of the acupuncture meridians, almost all of which end in the hands and feet. Applying pressure at points in the feet is akin to stimulating 'end-of-meridian' points. Reflexology is based on the same principle of stimulating and unblocking energy flows and the response to treatment is usually broadly similar, as is the range of disorders to which reflexology is applicable. Carried out by qualified reflexologists, sessions are normally given weekly.

colour therapy

Colour *can* be used to treat disease. Each colour in the spectrum has an effect on physical and mental well-being, and has its own energy that can interact with a patient in a positive way. For instance, red helps to increase energy levels (red clothing has been shown to increase blood pressure in a person), and will help to treat diseases such as circulatory problems and asthmatic coughs. Conversely, blue is calming and reduces blood pressure, and will assist in conditions such as epilepsy and diarrhoea. Orange might be used for anaemia and phobias; yellow for arthritis and acute or chronic eczema. Green is balancing, and will help heart problems and emotional trauma. Indigo is known as the colour for ear and eye disease, while violet is a relaxing colour, effective for kidney disease and sinusitis.

treatment

The obvious argument against the use of colour therapy for cats is that they do not see in colour, but it is not necessary to see the colour to derive benefit from it. It is the energy of the colour that is absorbed by the body – not the ability to visualize it – that is important, so colour therapy is perfectly applicable to cats.

The energy field of crystals and gems interacts with and works to stabilize the energy field of the patient, allowing natural healing to occur. The crystal or gem being used should be placed near the relevant 'chakra', or energy centre, of the body.

From the simple expedient of encouraging a dull, depressed cat to lie on a red blanket, to classic colour therapy in which coloured light is focused on the patient, colour can be beneficial. If you are using colour yourself, expose your cat to the same colour for up to two hours a day. Continue colour sessions for a week, or until you notice improvement.

A colour therapist, or chromopractitioner, may also be willing to work with animals, on referral from a vet; in this case, he or she will advise on the sessions required.

crystals and gems

The earliest use of crystals and gems as agents for healing can be traced back to Ancient Egypt. All crystals and gems, and indeed cats, vibrate at their own individual frequency, and the interaction between the energy field of the patient and that of the crystal will allow a stabilizing and healing action to take place. Different crystals and gems have different properties of healing. Amethyst, for example, can be a potent pain reliever (for both physical and

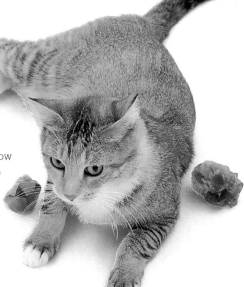

emotional pain). Ruby is beneficial for arthritic symptoms, Emerald for colitis (inflammation of the lining of the colon), and Citrine quartz will help to heal tissue damage after accidents and trauma.

treatment
If you are visiting a crystal therapist after referral from a vet, you will be given full instructions. If using crystals yourself, you can attach them to your cat's collar or a harness, which should be worn for two to three hours a day. Alternatively, place them on or around the body: they work particularly well at the body's traditional energy centres (chakras), such as at the top of the head, the throat and the stomach area. Leave the crystals in place for up to two hours a day.

    An alternative method of gem therapy is the use of liquid remedies. These are liquefied drops of crystals, minerals and gemstones, and are administered as for Bach flower essences (see pages 22–3), with one or two drops given daily by mouth or in drinking water. Like Bach flowers, the gem remedies are particularly applicable to mental and emotional disorders. For example, Sapphire is helpful for• hyperactivity and anxiety; Onyx might be useful for a very dominant, aggressive cat.

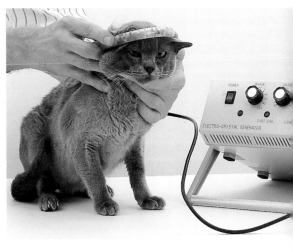

Electro-crystal therapy stabilizes energy imbalances. A sealed tube of crystals is placed on the affected area (or on the energy centre linked with that area) and then stimulated by an electric current.

electro-crystal therapy
Electro-crystal therapy (ECT) is a technique, pioneered by scientist Harry Oldfield, of diagnosing and treating energy imbalances in the body. It harnesses the known healing effect of crystals, but amplifies this by the use of electricity.

    In electro-crystal therapy, quartz crystals (immersed in a saline solution in a sealed tube) are stimulated by a small electric current administered at high frequency. The energy field that is created by the crystals under this electrical stimulation interacts with the energy field of the patient and works to stabilize energy imbalances. This allows healing of a wide range of illnesses, from bronchitis to back pain. The tube contains many different types of crystals, each of which has different healing effects. Varying the frequency of the electric current will stimulate the different crystal types in turn, to enhance systematically the healing action of the crystals that vibrate at each particular frequency.

treatment

This involves placing a sealed tube of crystals on the affected area (or on the energy centre that is linked with that area) and setting the appropriate frequency on a small generator connected to the tube. Sessions generally last from 10 to 20 minutes, depending on the severity of the problem and are usually undertaken at weekly intervals initially, progressing to longer intervals until the symptoms resolve completely. There is no discomfort while treatment is taking place, and no risk to the patient. Some qualified electro-crystal therapists are prepared to treat cats on referral from a vet.

healing

In a sense, healing – often known as spiritual or faith healing – is the purest form of treatment for illness, as it involves no pills, needles or equipment of any kind. The laying on of hands to heal disease is of ancient origin, and people with healing powers are acknowledged in all societies and cultures.

The source of the healing power is a matter of debate. Some healers believe that their abilities are divinely inspired, others have 'spirit guides', while some may have no fixed ideas about the derivation of their powers. However, all healers seem to feel that they act as a channel for healing energy, rather than actually carrying out the healing themselves. One particular form of hands-on healing, called Reiki, was developed by the Japanese theologian Mikao Usui who discovered in ancient Sanskrit writings a method of laying on hands that is now practised and taught worldwide.

Most reputable healers (in the UK) belong to the National Federation of Spiritual Healers, which operates in a strictly professional and ethical manner. The Federation has a code of conduct specifically regarding the treatment of animals. This was drawn up in conjunction with the Royal College of Veterinary Surgeons, and is an important guide to which all its members adhere.

Healing can help any illness or problem from which cats suffer, and is often effective with 'incurable' diseases such as cancer. Even if a cure is not achieved, animals almost always seem to feel better after healing sessions, with a reduction in pain or discomfort.

treatment

Healing sessions consist of a period of 10 to 20 minutes on average, during which the hands of the healer are held on or above the problem area. Many human patients report feeling a warm sensation in that part of the body. We obviously do not know whether animals feel the same effect, but most remain quiet and content during sessions. The number and frequency of healing sessions needed to help a patient will depend on the severity of the condition, but once a week until the condition is cured or under control is normal.

iridology

Iridology is primarily a diagnostic technique, rather than a therapy. The colour and shape of the iris in the eye, and its various marks, flecks and discolorations, reveal to the practised observer a mass of information regarding present health status, the location and type of any disease present, and any tendency towards future disease.

treatment

Different areas of the iris correspond to different parts of the body. Through careful examination of each eye under magnification, an iridologist will attempt to assess the exact location of the disorder, or where it may occur. The idea of this is to determine the root cause of the problem, so that it can be treated.

physiotherapy

Especially well-known for its undoubted ability to restore the use of damaged muscles, ligaments, tendons and bones, physiotherapy involves a range of techniques. In the UK there is an Association of Chartered Physiotherapists in Animal Therapy whose members are skilled in the specific treatment of pets, and many cats have benefited from their expert attention.

treatment

The most common form of treatment involves manipulation of the affected body part or parts. Other techniques may include using ultrasound, laser beams and even short-wave diathermy (a method of warming the muscles to accelerate the healing process).

The therapist to whom your cat is referred will suggest a schedule for treatment sessions, normally starting on a weekly basis. The total duration of treatment will depend on the progress of the disorder.

osteopathy

This is a manipulative therapy that has been practised for over 100 years. Although it is particularly effective for spinal problems in cats, osteopathy can also be used to treat joint and muscle disorders. To the lay person, osteopathy and chiropractic (see below) have much in common and may seem indistinguishable, but these two separate schools of manipulative therapy do in fact maintain that their techniques are quite different.

As far as feline patients are concerned, both osteopathy and chiropractic have proven invaluable in the case of chronic back problems and in helping to resolve persistent joint, muscle and nerve conditions. A number of osteopaths are now willing to treat cats, on referral from a vet, and many cats are a testament to the undoubted skills of these practitioners.

treatment

Osteopathy involves manipulation of the affected body parts. The therapist to whom your cat is referred will suggest a schedule for treatment sessions, normally starting on a weekly basis. The duration of treatment will depend on the progress of the disorder. In some instances one or two sessions of manipulation are sufficient; in other cases a longer course of treatment may be necessary.

chiropractic

Chiropractic is a manipulative therapy used in the treatment of muscular and joint disorders, especially those of the spine.

Although chiropractic was developed as a therapy for humans, and the anatomy of the cat is somewhat different from our own, the technique can be successfully applied to problems such as back pain, lameness and joint injuries. Some chiropractors are willing to treat cats, on referral from a vet.

treatment

Chiropractors use conventional investigative techniques – including X-ray pictures when necessary – to diagnose problems in their patients. With this form of treatment, manual stretching and massage are carried out in order to reduce muscle spasm and to ease joint stiffness. The chiropractor will advise on the length and frequency of treatment sessions, depending on the problem being treated. On average, three to 10 weekly sessions are required.

radionics

This is another natural therapy based on the energy pattern of an individual, and on the belief that a disruption in this pattern is a reflection of the disease process. Radionics is a method of identifying a change in the energy pattern, and of finding ways of correcting it.

Cats appear to respond well to radionics, and some practitioners of this therapy are beginning to specialize in treating them. A radionics practitioner may also suggest the use of additional therapies such as homoeopathy, physiotherapy or osteopathy.

treatment

A practitioner of radionics will take a clump of fur, or another small part of body tissue, from the cat: this is often known as the 'witness'. (On the principle that all parts of the body will reflect the energy disruption, a small sample of fur will be quite sufficient for an analysis to be made.) The sample is scanned by a radionic instrument, which measures energy patterns and isolates the problem area in the body. Other radionic instruments then 'broadcast' healing energy back to the patient, to correct the imbalance and to stimulate healing to occur.

A radionics practitioner can operate at some distance from the patient and, because treatment takes place via the 'witness', does not necessarily even need to see him or her. However, a full history of the illness, together with relevant information about any previous medical problems and a general description of the patient, are required.

The duration of treatment will vary according to the type of problem and the cat concerned. A recently acquired illness may improve within a few days; a chronic problem may take weeks or months.

dowsing

Rather more of a diagnostic tool than a therapy, it is interesting to note that the age-old art of dowsing has an ancient application in medicine. Although most of us have heard about and probably seen the art of dowsing for water, it is less commonly known that dowsing can be used to discover sites of disease in the body, and even to learn which remedy or remedies will be curative for that disease.

treatment

By noting the oscillation of a pendulum held over a patient, an expert dowser can find out much information that may be useful in assessing the type and extent of disease, and the therapy that may be indicated.

a healthy life

This section is dedicated to the principle that prevention is better than cure. It concentrates on measures that will help to keep your cat fit and well, and examines the external factors that affect health.

your cat's environment

The main reason for any general improvement in health is usually due to a better quality of living standards: clean drinking water, efficient sewage disposal, adequate ventilation, better hygiene, less-crowded living conditions and a good diet. These environmental factors, far more than any modern medicines, reduce the risks of disease and enable us to live longer.

A safe, healthy environment is equally important for our cats, in whom there recently appears to have been a great increase in chronic conditions such as disease of the immune system, eczema and sinusitis. One reason for this may be the increasing pollution of the environment: of the air, of water, and of the land. The continuing over-use of pesticides, fertilizers and other chemicals on farmland, and the factory waste pumped into rivers and the air, is placing a burden both on our immune systems and on those of our pets, particularly those who are prone to chronic illness. It therefore follows that we should be conscious of the following potential dangers in the environment – both outdoors and indoors.

air

Do not expose a cat with any degree of bronchitis, or any other respiratory disease, to cigarette smoke. Adequate ventilation at all times is also vital.

A cat who has a history of coughs or other respiratory symptoms may benefit from the use of an ionizer, which will help to keep the air fresh and clean. You should consider a humidifier if the air is very dry, especially when central heating is in operation, as dry air is very harmful to the delicate tissues of the respiratory tract.

Try to reduce the volume of any chemicals used around the house that your cat may absorb, such as room-freshener sprays, hair sprays and fly sprays. These sprays all contain substances that may be harmful to pets.

A humidifier is a simple device, used to counter the effects of central heating and very dry air. Alternatively, place a bowl of water near a radiator – this will help to maintain moisture levels.

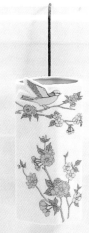

Some cats seem to suffer from a syndrome similar to our hay fever, so reducing the time allowed outside on days with high pollen counts is worthwhile.

water

I firmly believe that tap water can aggravate health problems in some cats. The chemicals added to tap water – such as chlorine – as well as pollutants that may be

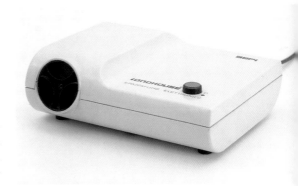

present, appear to act as a precipitating factor in the progression of eczema and other inflammatory disorders. Cats certainly seem to prefer – and benefit from – drinking filtered or mineral water instead of ordinary tap water.

Drinking and feeding bowls should be ceramic or stainless steel, as the chemicals from plastic may leach out into water or food.

Ionizers can be expensive, but are a worthwhile investment. They will help to keep the air fresh and clean, and can be beneficial for a cat who suffers from respiratory problems.

land

Try to avoid allowing your cat to roam in or near fields that have recently been sprayed with fertilizers or other chemicals. Skin irritation can result, as can itchiness after running through certain grasses in the springtime. During winter, try to prevent your cat from walking on roads or pavements that have been gritted and salted: exposure to treated roads can cause severe foot inflammation.

It is said that nomadic people, and the animals who travel with them, seldom suffer from chronic illness. One theory for this is that many of us who stay in one place for long periods are exposed to 'geopathic stress'. This phenomenon is said to be a result of natural radiation rising up through the Earth and being distorted by electromagnetic fields created by underground streams, mineral deposits and fault lines. The distortion interacts with our own energy field – and that of our cats – to create chronic illness.

I know of several families where persistent illness was evident in both the family members and their pets, and for whom a move of house seemed to bring a new lease of life to all concerned. I am not suggesting moving home whenever chronic disease occurs, but persistent illness in an entire household for no apparent reason could suggest the possibility of geopathic stress as a factor.

lifestyle

Providing the perfect environment for your cat will be pointless unless he or she also leads a healthy life. While it is not practicable to take a cat out for exercise, you should encourage play and activity in the house. Kittens will naturally play with many objects, and older cats can usually be persuaded to do so.

Letting a cat out will not necessarily result in exercise, as many cats will just sit still for long periods. It may also not be safe: you must decide whether to allow your cat the freedom to go outdoors according to the amount of local traffic and the presence of any other hazards such as fierce dogs or, more probably, fierce cats. Your own cat's personality will also be a factor in the lifestyle that he or she leads: some cats seem perfectly happy to lead an indoor life; others appear to become frustrated and even depressed.

hygiene

Grooming is something that most people imagine cats do for themselves. Certainly, short-haired individuals need little attention (although they may appreciate and enjoy gentle brushing), but long-haired breeds need frequent and thorough grooming as their coats are prone to tangle and mat. On several occasions over the years I have had to anaesthetize and completely shave a Persian cat whose fur had become one solid mat from lack of grooming.

You should also carry out regular health-checks on your cat. Look at his or her eyes, ears and nose for any signs of inflammation or discharge, and check the teeth for discoloration or tartar formation. Take note of any abnormal smells coming from the ears, breath or skin. Move your hands over the cat's body and feel for any unusual lumps or swellings, and check the skin for signs of fleas or other parasites. As you get to know what your cat looks, smells and feels like, you will notice any abnormality in its early stages.

A cat's bedding should be frequently laundered. If an individual suffers from a persistent skin condition, an allergic reaction to the bedding may be the cause, and the bedding may need to be replaced. Your vet can carry out skin tests to determine an allergy of this kind.

nutrition

Take one demanding cat, one overworked, tired owner, one supermarket shelf marked 'pet foods' and who could resist reaching for a bag of dried food, or a convenient can? That is, until a problem arises. Take one distressed cat with diarrhoea, one equally distressed owner and one holistic vet, and the advice may well be to resist the 'convenient can' temptation.

commercial cat foods

There is no doubt that many health disorders in cats can be prevented or cured by paying attention to the diet. So what is in that can or that bag of food that may be less than positive for our pets?

Water Many canned foods have a water content of up to 80 per cent. Apart from the fact that the water itself – if not filtered or pure – could be potentially harmful, a high water content can predispose some cats to loose bowel movements.

Additives Most canned foods also contain artificial flavouring and colouring. However, a good food should be tasty enough for a cat to eat without the addition of flavouring and, as cats do not see colour in the same way that we do, any colouring added is for our benefit, not theirs. Sodium nitrate, for instance, imparts a nice rosy colour to the food, but it has been linked to disease in pets.

BHA and BHT are two other additives that may produce liver and kidney problems and are used as additives in some foods. Other contaminants, such as hormones and antibiotics, could be found if the meat has come from intensively reared livestock. Salt and sugar at unacceptably high levels occasionally occur, especially in semi-moist cat foods (those with up to 50 per cent water). There is no need for any sugar in cat food, and salt levels of over 2 per cent are unnecessary.

Labelling Reading the label of a prepared cat food may be confusing. For instance, different brands of food may contain the same level of protein, but not all protein is the same: the protein obtained from meat by-products – which may include items such as feathers, hair and even leather – may be less nutritious than those from 'real' meat. These different types of protein have different biological uses (not all proteins are as useful as others), and some are more difficult to digest.

For such reasons, it is very difficult to compare like with like when comparing cat foods, or to calculate nutritional value. This is not to say that manufacturers purposefully produce sub-standard food for cats, but the ingredients used may not always be the best available.

When using proprietary foods, you should therefore look for quality ingredients, with as few by-products, colourings, flavourings and preservatives as possible, and low sugar and salt levels. You may prefer to use dried foods, to which you can add your own water (rather than paying for it in the tin!), but there are some good-quality canned foods available. If you do decide to use dried foods and to add your own water, you should ensure that the water is either filtered or mineral if at all possible (see page 39).

Above all, the food must be palatable, as there is no point in trying to force your cat to eat a diet that he or she does not enjoy. If you do so, the cat may well try to scavenge food from elsewhere, and will ruin the balanced diet that you are trying to feed.

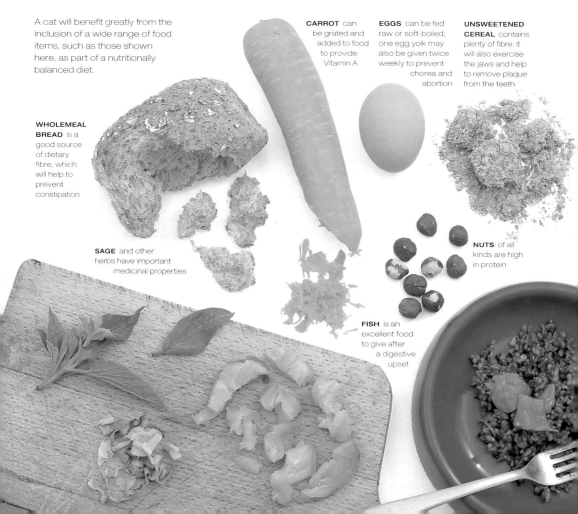

A cat will benefit greatly from the inclusion of a wide range of food items, such as those shown here, as part of a nutritionally balanced diet.

CARROT can be grated and added to food to provide Vitamin A

EGGS can be fed raw or soft-boiled; one egg yolk may also be given twice weekly to prevent chorea and abortion

UNSWEETENED CEREAL contains plenty of fibre. It will also exercise the jaws and help to remove plaque from the teeth

WHOLEMEAL BREAD is a good source of dietary fibre, which will help to prevent constipation

SAGE and other herbs have important medicinal properties

NUTS of all kinds are high in protein

FISH is an excellent food to give after a digestive upset

a vegetarian diet

Is it possible to feed a cat safely on a vegetarian diet? This question is sometimes asked by vegetarian owners who cannot face the idea of preparing meat for their charges. The answer is that, unfortunately, cats are what is known as obligate carnivores: in other words, they must have a source of animal protein in their diet.

This is because two nutrients found almost solely in animal tissue are required by cats to stay healthy. The first is arachadonic acid, one of the essential fatty acids. The substances known as the EFAs are needed by the body for normal kidney function, and to maintain normal healthy skin, and they are also vital for healthy reproduction. Cats need arachadonic acid as one of their EFAs, and, as it is almost never found in plants, an animal source of food is necessary.

Similarly, the amino acid taurine, which is derived almost totally from animal tissue, is vital for normal retinal function – a deficiency in taurine will cause blindness.

CABBAGE should be grated and fed raw to preserve its vitamin content

Cats must therefore be fed some real meat in their diets, or be given a vegetarian diet supplemented by the missing nutrients. The latter option can be taken, and prepared vegetarian cat foods are now on the market, but my opinion is that cats evolved as meat eaters, and that to deny them their natural carnivorous habits is to impose our human morals on their instinctive feeding behaviour.

a home-made diet

Having looked at why it might be better not to feed your cat processed foods, what is the alternative? There is, in my view, no single perfect diet. Variations in size, age and metabolism, and in simple taste preference, mean that a diet that suits one cat will not necessarily suit another.

It seems sensible, when feeding a natural, home-produced diet, to try to keep it as close to the food intake of a wild cat as is practical. A wild cat will kill its prey and then eat it raw, often starting with the internal organs (such as the intestines, liver and heart), and saving the meat and bones for later. The intestines will contain the grains and other vegetable matter eaten by the prey animal, and are therefore a useful source of these items.

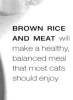

BROWN RICE AND MEAT will make a healthy, balanced meal that most cats should enjoy

In most cases, it is unlikely that we will send our cats out to hunt for food, although some do so for themselves to a greater or lesser extent. However, a diet that is reasonably similar to that of the wild cat is ideal in principle. If you do not like the idea of feeding raw meat, grains and vegetables to your cat, a modified version may be more acceptable and is still very healthy. The main priority is to achieve a balanced, nutritious diet, and this should be composed of the following items.

Meat This should constitute approximately 60 per cent of the total meal. Raw meat is ideal – especially if organically produced – as cooking will denature and destroy some of the nutrients. The exceptions to this rule are raw pork and rabbit, which may contain parasites and so should be cooked. However, avoid overcooking, in order to retain as many of the nutrients of the meat as possible. It is a good idea to give some of the meat in reasonably sized chunks, as it is good exercise for your cat's jaws to chew at large pieces of meat.

Some fish (without bones) and white meat (chicken or turkey) should be included as part of the meat content, as a diet that is composed mainly of red meat can be too rich for some cats. Offal – to imitate the consumption of the internal organs in the wild – should also be included. Heart, tripe, kidneys and liver in small amounts are all suitable (raw liver should never be given in large quantities, as your cat could have an overdose of Vitamin A).

Other ingredients The remaining 40 per cent of a cat's diet should include vegetables, fruit, pulses, nuts and grains. A variety of these foods is suitable, including cooked brown rice, grated raw vegetables such as carrots and courgettes, unsweetened cereals and fruit. Grains and pulses will be digested better if they are cooked beforehand, simulating the fact that the vegetable matter in the body of a wild cat's prey will already be partially digested.

additional foods

A natural, nutritionally balanced diet for a cat should also contain some or all of the following foods, given in the quantities suggested here.

Eggs Most cats will eat eggs raw or soft-boiled. One egg per week will be adequate.

Live yoghurt This is not only a nutritious food in itself, but the natural bacteria that it contains will help your cat's digestive tract to function efficiently: 5 ml (1 tsp) daily is ideal.

Milk Although many cats enjoy milk, you should only give it in small quantities as it is not a natural food. In addition, some cats have difficulty in digesting the lactose in milk, and may have diarrhoea.

Natural oils Add 5 ml (1 tsp) of sesame, sunflower or safflower oil to food once or twice weekly to help to balance your cat's diet.

when to feed
Once-daily feeding is suitable for a cat whose digestion seems to cope with occasional large meals – as it would do in the wild. However, most cats seem to thrive better on two or three small meals a day.

how much to feed
The age, breed, size, resting metabolic rate and lifestyle of a cat will all affect his or her feeding requirements. A combination of common sense and, if necessary, advice from your vet should indicate the volume of food that your cat needs. From then onwards, simply watch his or her weight and energy. If your cat is becoming overweight and seems lethargic, cut back on the calories; if his or her weight decreases, increase the amount of food. If any weight loss persists, or a weight increase is not controlled by a reduction in food intake, you should seek further veterinary advice.

Obesity is one of the main factors involved in the onset of arthritis, diabetes, liver problems, skin troubles and heart disorders in middle-aged and older cats, yet no cat is born to be overweight. If obesity is a problem with your cat, your vet will help you to plan and maintain a programme of weight reduction. Without doubt, adopting a natural diet as described earlier will help.

dietary changes
If you intend to alter your cat's diet, never try to do so suddenly as this may cause a bout of diarrhoea (see page 101). Always introduce any new foods gradually, allowing about 10 days to complete the full changeover, as any sudden change may cause a digestive upset. Remember too that growing kittens, pregnant and elderly cats all have different nutritional requirements: the guidelines given in this book are for an average, healthy, adult cat.

Always consult your vet before implementing any drastic change in diet, especially if your cat has any ongoing health problems, or a past history of recurrent illness.

supplements

Certain dietary supplements can help to overcome any possible deficiencies in your cat's diet. There are two types: nutritional supplements such as vitamins and minerals, which balance the diet or add 'missing' ingredients; and health supplements, which can enhance the immune system or help to fight infection, but may have no direct nutritional benefit.

nutritional supplements

In theory, if an adult cat is eating a balanced diet of high-quality ingredients no other supplements should be necessary, but in practice even a home-produced diet may contain ingredients that are lower in vitamins or minerals than is ideal for the maintenance of optimum fitness and well-being. Certainly, commercial cat foods – even with added vitamins and minerals – may still lose some of their vitamin content during processing or storage. Young, pregnant, ill or old cats in particular may have special needs for certain supplements. Those that I find have real merit are as follows.

Kelp This powder is produced from seaweed, and is rich in minerals (especially iodine). It complements vitamin-rich brewer's yeast to provide an optimum multi-vitamin and multi-mineral combination from natural sources. The mineral content of kelp helps to maintain the efficient functioning of many body processes, including red-blood-cell production, and hormonal and metabolic reactions. Give 1 tsp daily.

Vitamin C This vitamin is well-known for its action in accelerating the healing of damaged tissue, and for its role in maintaining healthy immune and circulatory systems, and strong bones and joints. There is also evidence that it may help to minimize the risk of cancer. Cats produce some natural Vitamin C, but a supplement is a good idea, especially as this vitamin is not stored in the body. Give 250 mg daily.

Vitamin E This vitamin helps to fight infection and disease. It is an antioxidant, and helps to preserve the activity of Vitamin A and fatty acids in food. Wheatgerm oil is a good source of Vitamin E, and promotes a good, glossy coat. Vitamin E is also available as capsules.

Be sure to use a natural Vitamin E, rather than a synthetic form (look for 'd-alpha tocopherol' on the label), as most vitamins from natural sources are absorbed better by the body and appear to have a more positive effect than their synthetic counterparts. Approximately 50 iu (international units) per day is a suitable dosage rate.

Cod-liver oil Apart from its invaluable effect in helping to prevent and treat the symptoms of arthritis, and in promoting a healthy skin and coat, the Vitamins A and D in cod-liver oil are active in the body in myriad ways. Eyesight, tooth formation, nervous tissue and bones and joints are all parts of the body that Vitamins A and D assist in developing and in maintaining normal function. Vitamin A is also an antioxidant and combats the effects of chemicals and pollutants.

A suitable dosage rate of cod-liver oil is one 300 mg capsule daily. This provides about 600 iu Vitamin A and 60 iu Vitamin D per capsule, depending on the brand used. Cod-liver oil must never be over-used, because excessive amounts of Vitamin A can damage bones and joints. It is sensible to give cod-liver oil to a cat intermittently rather than continuously: one week in four is a good ratio.

health supplements

The following supplements can be positive adjuncts to a nutritionally balanced and supplemented diet. In addition to those described here, there is an enormous range of other supplements that are claimed to have health-giving properties for cats, such as ginseng, ginkgo and propolis. Any or all of these may well be beneficial, but I have included supplements of which I have personal experience.

Chlorella This green alga is rich in vitamins and minerals. It increases energy and stamina, as well as promoting the production of red blood cells and assisting rapid healing of damaged tissue. It also seems to strengthen the immune system, neutralize environmental toxins and enhance the destruction of cancer cells.

Chlorella is available in tablet form and also as a powdered supplement. The normal dosage rate for a cat is 1 g per day. Reports from the owners of regular users talk of improved skin and coat condition, reduction in bad breath, fewer digestive upsets and less incidence of disease.

Royal jelly This is a substance secreted by worker bees to feed the growing larvae of the queen bee. A larva fed on royal jelly will itself become a queen, growing larger, living 50 times longer than a normal bee, and laying up to 2000 eggs per day.

Luckily, royal jelly does not have quite such a dramatic effect on cats, but it is a valuable health supplement. It seems to have a stabilizing action on certain metabolic processes in the body – especially those linked to skin and coat condition, energy, appetite and temperament. Royal jelly also has a peculiar capacity to increase the energy levels of a dull and depressed cat, yet it will help to calm a nervous, excitable and hyperactive cat. It can improve a poor appetite, but will not encourage over-eating. In virtually all cases, it will noticeably improve skin and coat condition.

Supplements added to a cat's diet can have positive health-giving results.

GARLIC is well-known as 'nature's disinfectant', and makes an invaluable health supplement

Fresh royal jelly gives much better results than the freeze-dried version. A dosage rate of 100 mg daily is recommended.

Garlic As well as being a specific herbal remedy for ailments such as chronic respiratory disease, garlic can be given to a cat as a general supplement because of its wide-ranging action in the body. Garlic works as an anti-infective agent, helps to reduce the level of parasites in cats (internal and external), and stimulates normal digestive processes.

DRIED YEAST is a good source of B-complex and other vitamins and minerals

Ideally, $\frac{1}{3}$ fresh clove of garlic should be given daily. Most cats will accept this, especially if finely chopped or grated and mixed with food. Alternatively, garlic capsules are acceptable: 2 mg of essential garlic oil seems to give the same effect as $\frac{1}{3}$ clove of fresh garlic. Odourless garlic capsules are also available, but I have found that these are less successful in keeping parasites such as fleas at bay.

Dried yeast This is good natural source of B-complex and other vitamins and minerals. Brewer's yeast is the preferred variety. The B group of vitamins has many functions in the body, including that of helping to fight disease. Give $\frac{1}{4}$ tsp daily.

administering tablets

Knowing the dosage rate of a tablet is one thing, but giving a tablet can be quite another. If your cat hates taking tablets, here are a few tips that are more likely to achieve success at the first attempt, and therefore to cause your cat – and you – the minimum of distress and anxiety. A special syringe known as a 'pill giver' is a very useful tool for administrating tablets. It also prevents the possibility of contaminating tablets by touching them, which is particularly important when using homoeopathic remedies (see page 15).

using a pill giver

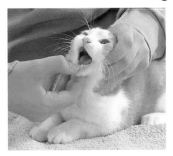

I Shake the tablet from its container into the syringe. Hold the cat's head with one hand, with your thumb and fingers on either side of his or her face. Gently tilt the head upwards. Use the thumb of your other hand to draw down the lower jaw, and then squeeze gently with the first hand to keep the jaws apart.

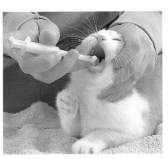

2 Still holding the cat's head tilted upwards, take the syringe in your free hand and, holding it over the centre of the tongue, depress the plunger to release the tablet into the mouth. Your aim should be to drop the tablet as far back into the cat's mouth as possible, as this will make it more difficult to spit out.

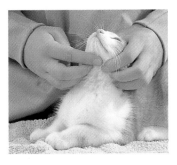

3 Allow the mouth to close, but keep the cat's head tilted upwards. Using one or more fingers, gently rub down the cat's throat in order to encourage swallowing. Alternatively, if you are giving a 'soft' homoeopathic tablet that does not need to be swallowed (see page 15), simply keep the cat's mouth closed to allow absorption.

common

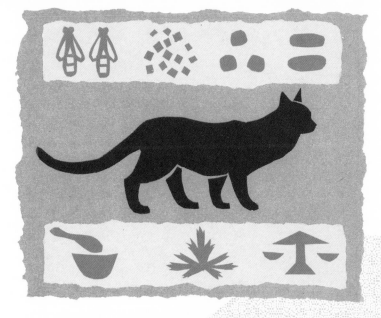

diseases
and conditions

This section covers the main diseases and problems that cats may experience, and the natural medicines that can be used to help to relieve the symptoms or to promote a cure. However, the advice given here is not a substitute for veterinary attention. Any condition that causes your cat to appear seriously unwell, persists for more than a day or two, or has unusual symptoms, needs veterinary advice as soon as possible. Never take risks with your cat's health, and never try to avoid using conventional medicine simply because you prefer natural therapies. Conventional drugs have their drawbacks, but in some cases – for example, when antibiotics are used to treat an acute infection – they can be life-savers.

Although you should never attempt to treat an acute condition solely with natural medicines unless you have been advised to do so by a vet, it is perfectly permissible and indeed a good idea to use them in an emergency while you are waiting for veterinary assistance. Minor problems – small cuts and bruises, digestive upsets, itchy skin, and so on – can be safely treated, but if the condition persists you must take your cat to the vet.

This part of the book is designed to help you to understand how natural medicines work, and to make using them easy and effective. It begins with vital instructions on what to do for your cat in an emergency situation. This is followed by information on a wide range of common diseases and conditions to affect cats, which are ordered according to body systems: for example, sprains and strains will be found in the musculo-skeletal system, and gingivitis in the digestive system. Each disease or condition has a brief explanation of what it is, how it is caused and what the typical symptoms may be, followed by advice on the natural remedies that will help to treat it.

For information on the dosage and administration of the remedies, refer to the *natural therapies* section (see pages 8–37).

emergencies

When a serious accident or other emergency occurs, it is easy to panic. Clear thinking is invaluable at times of crisis, and this will only be possible if you are prepared. Familiarize yourself with the following advice so that, in the event of an emergency, you will know how to care for your cat in the best way possible, as quickly as possible. Natural medicines should be an integral part of your plan, but first aid may be required initially. Do not give an injured cat anything to eat or drink, unless on veterinary advice, in case surgery is required.

emergency action

Keep a clear head and take the following steps in the event of an accident or other emergency.

assess the situation

Check whether the injured cat is conscious, is still breathing and has a heartbeat, using the following techniques:

• A conscious cat will react to a noise, or if you pinch the skin between his or her toes, and should blink if you pass a hand in front of the eyes.
• To check breathing, watch for rising and falling chest movements, or hold a piece of tissue paper or a feather in front of the cat's nose.
• To feel for a heartbeat, press gently on the chest behind the elbow.

prevent further harm

The action needed should be obvious: for example, if the cat has been electrocuted, turn off the power supply immediately, *before* handling the cat; if the cat has been burned, move him or her away from the heat source; direct traffic away from an accident site, or carefully move the cat away, using a makeshift stretcher such as a board or blanket.

contact your vet

Carry out any necessary life-saving procedures first (see opposite), then contact a vet as soon as possible – have your vet's telephone number available at all times – and make transport arrangements.

restrain the cat

Even a normally gentle cat who is in pain may bite or lash out. To avoid this, wrap him or her in a towel or thick blanket. If the cat is loose, approach slowly and quietly; if the cat seems to be badly injured, cover him or her with a blanket or aluminium foil to keep in body heat.

first aid

After taking emergency action, first aid is the next step. The basic techniques described here are not difficult to learn, and could save your cat's life in the minutes before veterinary help arrives.

clear the airway

If the cat is not breathing, or is choking, check for obstructions to the airway. Put the cat on his or her side, open the jaws and gently pull the tongue forward. Remove any debris in the nose, mouth or throat.

carry out artificial respiration

If the cat is not breathing but there is a heartbeat, carry out artificial respiration. Close the cat's mouth and, keeping it closed, gently blow into the nostrils until you see the chest rise. Then let the lungs deflate naturally, before beginning the process again. Repeat this procedure 15 times per minute, or until breathing starts spontaneously.

carry out heart massage

If there is no breathing or heartbeat, alternate 15-second spells of artificial respiration with 15-second periods of heart massage. To do this, use the fingers and thumb of one hand to squeeze the chest wall, compressing the chest strongly, then release. Repeat as frequently as possible (at least once, or preferably twice per second). Alternate heart massage with artificial respiration until the heart restarts, and then continue with artificial respiration until breathing restarts.

control bleeding

• If a wound is bleeding uncontrollably, apply pressure at the point of bleeding. Any padding is suitable – sterility is not essential in an emergency. Apply absorbent padding, overlaid by as many layers of firm bandaging material as necessary, until the bleeding stops.

• If an object – such as a piece of glass – is protruding from the wound, do not try to remove it as you may well cause further damage. Instead, make a ring-shaped pad by twisting a length of material into a doughnut shape, and then place this around the wound before gently bandaging the pad in position.

• Only bandage a wound in the case of severe bleeding. Do not apply a tourniquet above the bleeding point: this can obstruct the blood supply to healthy tissue and cause permanent damage. Place a rolled- up towel under the cat's hindquarters to assist blood flow to the heart and head.

wounds

The inquisitive nature of cats seems to predispose them to accidents, but, luckily, they are often capable of surprisingly rapid recovery. Road-traffic accidents are by far the most common cause of serious injuries. Other common accidents include falling out of trees or windows, being cut by empty food cans, and getting tails shut in doors. Carry out first aid initially (see page 53), then make use of the valuable assistance of natural medicines.

aromatherapy

Lavender and Terebinth may be massaged in the region of (but not on the actual site of) a wound.

homoeopathy

Arnica (acute dosage) is the perfect tissue-trauma remedy. This will prevent or minimize bruising, help to stop bleeding and heal damaged and traumatized tissue speedily. Calendula (lotion or ointment) may be applied directly to a wound or abrasion to promote healing.

herbal medicine

An infusion of Blackberry may be applied directly to the wound. Geranium leaves can also be wrapped around a wound or bruising to aid healing (see opposite, above).

Bach flowers

Rescue Remedy, given by mouth in single drops, is helpful for the shock resulting from an injury.

minor therapies

biochemical tissue salts

Ferr. phos. (acute dosage) may be administered by mouth, or applied directly to the affected area.

homoeopathy for injuries

Nine Lives was a young kitten whose name was certainly a self-fulfilling prophecy. When I first met him he had already used up several 'lives', and this time I found him hobbling into my surgery on three legs. The injured limb had been trapped in a car door, after the kitten had somehow managed to wriggle out of his carrying basket. Luckily the leg was not fractured, but simply bruised and lacerated.

Nine Lives's owner was a keen gardener – particularly proud of her Geraniums – and I pressed her horticultural efforts into service. As well as giving treatment with homoeopathic Arnica for the trauma, I asked her to tape some Geranium leaves around the damaged leg, and to change them daily. Within a week the leg had healed, and Nine Lives was out and about, looking for more ways of living up to his name.

Chinese medicine

Apply the juice of crushed chive leaves and roots to the site of an abrasion or laceration to speed healing. This will also help to reduce the bruising.

crystals and gems

Pearl (liquid-gem remedy) may be given by mouth as single drops. Citrine quartz will also aid healing.

wrapping a wound

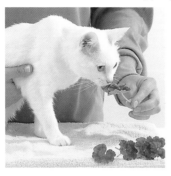 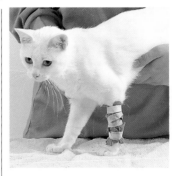

1 Geranium leaves can be wrapped around a wound to aid healing. Pick as many fresh leaves as necessary to cover the area of the wound.

2 Place the leaves over the wound, securing them with medical adhesive tape (be very careful not to apply this too tightly). Change the leaves daily.

bites and stings
Dogs and other cats are the main culprits of bite wounds. Bites can become infected, and should be carefully cleaned with a veterinary antiseptic solution before being treated as described below. Spring and autumn are the peak danger periods for stings (kittens in particular love chasing insects). If the area around a bite or sting is very hot and red, bathe it with cold water, or apply a cold compress such as an ice pack or a bag of frozen peas.

aromatherapy
Lavender will be soothing if massaged gently around a bite or a sting, but should not be applied directly to an open wound.

homoeopathy
Apis mel. is ideal for treating an insect sting, especially if the area is swollen and red; Hypericum will help to relieve a painful bite or sting; and Arnica may be used for a bite that has resulted in an open wound and bruising (all in acute dosage).

herbal medicine
An infusion of Rosemary can be used to bathe the area surrounding a bite or a sting.

Bach flowers
Rescue Remedy will help to calm and quieten a frightened or distressed cat.

minor therapies
biochemical tissue salts
Nat. mur. can be applied locally to the site of an insect sting; Ferr. phos. to a bite wound (in acute dosage).

haemorrhaging

Severe bleeding may be the result of a road-traffic or other accident, a puncture wound or a dog or cat bite. Although the feline body – as the human body – has an effective blood-clotting mechanism, if a major blood vessel becomes damaged or even severed in an accident, a life-threatening haemorrhage may occur. In the case of haemorrhaging, the first step is to carry out appropriate emergency treatment (see page 53) in order to prevent an excessive loss of blood. Once any immediate threat to the cat's life has been resolved, treatment with the following remedies will help to stop further bleeding, and will reduce pain and shock.

aromatherapy

Lavender can be gently massaged near the site of the haemorrhage (but never directly at the source of the bleeding).

homoeopathy

Arnica (acute dosage) is a superb remedy for helping to stop a serious haemorrhage as rapidly as possible. Hamamelis (acute dosage) is useful for the slow seepage of blood that is dark and venous (as compared with the acute 'spurting' of bright-red blood that is a telltale sign of damage to an artery). Hamamelis is also a good remedy for a haematoma, which is a haemorrhage that occurs inside the earflap (see page 67).

herbal medicine

If the compresses and bandages used to apply pressure at the point of haemorrhage are first soaked in an infusion of Rosemary, the bleeding is likely to cease more quickly. An infusion of Meadowsweet can also be used in this way (either alone or in combination with the Rosemary).

Bach flowers

Rescue Remedy is ideal for reducing the shock associated with severe bleeding following an accident, and should be given as single drops by mouth (one drop every five minutes).

minor therapies

biochemical tissue salts

Ferr. phos. (acute dosage) is a good remedy to control haemorrhaging. The tablets may be administered by mouth or, alternatively, may be powdered and then applied directly to the site of the bleeding (the best way to do this without the risk of contaminating the tablets is to fold them in a clean sheet of paper before crushing them).

Chinese medicine

Eggshells – powdered and applied to the bleeding point – will promote rapid clotting of the blood. A piece of baked, dried chicken will have the same effect, should you happen to have any of this to hand!

crystals and gems

Pearl (liquid-gem remedy) may be given by mouth in single drops.

collapse and shock

A cat who is in shock may be unconscious or semi-conscious, with pale or bluish gums and shallow breathing. Possible causes could be involvement in a road-traffic accident, electrocution, a diabetic coma, or even heart failure. Heart 'attacks' and coronary heart disease are rare in cats, but other heart defects will occasionally cause collapse. So too will anaphylactic shock: an acute allergic reaction to stings, drugs or (in rare instances) to food. Give first aid immediately (see page 53), and keep the cat warm until veterinary help arrives.

homoeopathy

Aconite is helpful in all cases of shock, and can be safely powdered into the mouth of an unconscious patient. Carbo vegetabilis is ideal for a cat who has collapsed but is still conscious and shows a desire for fresh air. Ver. alb. should be given to a cat who has collapsed and is very cold, with bluish gums; this will also help to reduce diarrhoea, a common accompanying symptom. All three remedies should be given in acute dosage.

herbal medicine

An infusion of Elder blossom is suitable for a victim recovering from shock. However, this should never be given to an unconscious or semi-conscious patient, as it could be inhaled rather than swallowed.

Bach flowers

Rescue Remedy is recommended for treating a cat who is in shock and has collapsed. Apply single drops of the remedy directly into the mouth of an unconscious cat every five minutes.

minor therapies

biochemical tissue salts
Nat. sulph. (acute dosage) can be powdered into the mouth of an unconscious cat.

crystals and gems
Pearl (liquid-gem remedy) can be given by mouth, as single drops, to a conscious or unconscious cat.

using Rescue Remedy

Vets just have to get used to the telephone ringing at unsocial hours. At 3 am the urge to ignore the summons is particularly strong, but on this occasion – as usual – I managed to put duty before instinct and answer the call. 'Chairman is unconscious' was the brief message. On questioning, this was expanded to the information that the cat involved (Chairman Meeow) had been hit by a car, had struggled home, but was now lying unconscious.

While I was on my way, I advised the owner to give one drop of Rescue Remedy every five minutes. When I arrived, Chairman – by now fully recovered – ran to greet me. He must have received just a glancing blow from the car and suffered only shock, which the Rescue Remedy had resolved. Gratefully, I returned to bed.

poisoning

If you believe that your cat has swallowed a poison, your first thought may be to make him or her sick. However, if the poison is a strong acid or alkali, or is oil-based (see below), this may be harmful. It is also dangerous to make an unconscious cat vomit. If you are certain that the poison is not acidic, alkaline or oil-based, induce vomiting with a small piece of washing soda (sodium carbonate) or a concentrated salt solution (2.5 ml [½ tsp] every five minutes, until vomiting occurs). A cat can also ingest poison by licking a substance on his or her fur, so remove any tar, oil, paraffin, petrol, creosote or paint immediately with warm water and liquid detergent.

acid, alkali and oil-based poisons

battery acid

bleach

dishwasher detergent

drain cleaner

motor oil

oven cleaner

paint thinners and stripper

paraffin, petrol

polish

toilet cleaner

washing detergent

Give bicarbonate of soda, egg white or vegetable oil (acid poisons); egg white, vinegar or lemon juice (alkali poisons); and natural remedies as advised (oil-based poisons).

other poisons

anti-freeze

aspirin and paracetamol

insecticide

mouse, rat and slug bait

Induce vomiting if the poison has been recently swallowed.

aromatherapy

Mint given by gentle massage will aid recovery from poisoning.

homoeopathy

Aconite is helpful for the shock associated with poisoning. Nux vomica is particularly useful following consumption of poisonous plants and Strychnine-based poisons. Ver. alb. may be given where poisoning has resulted in collapse, a cold body and diarrhoea. All three remedies should be given in acute dosage.

herbal medicine

An infusion of Hyssop will assist recovery, but should not be given to an unconscious cat.

Bach flowers

Rescue Remedy administered by mouth will help to overcome shock.

minor therapies

Chinese medicine

Honey may be given by mouth, at the rate of 2.5 ml (½ tsp) every 15 minutes for four hours.

burns

Burns are generally caused by heat or boiling liquids, but electrical burns sometimes occur, as do caustic burns resulting from contact with certain chemicals. Do not apply butter or vegetable oil to a burn as – contrary to popular belief – this will not be helpful, but do bathe a burn liberally with cold water before applying a cold compress such as an ice pack or a bag of frozen peas.

aromatherapy

Lavender and Rosemary can be massaged around the site of a burn, but not directly on to the burn itself.

homoeopathy

Cantharis (acute dosage) may be used to relieve the pain of burns and scalds of all kinds.

Bach flowers

Rescue Remedy, given in single drops by mouth, will help to alleviate shock and fright.

minor therapies

biochemical tissue salts

Kali mur. (acute dosage) may be given by mouth; alternatively, the tablets may be dissolved in cold water (two tablets in 5 ml [1 tsp] water) to make a lotion, and then applied directly to the area of the burn.

Chinese medicine

Freshly pressed ginger juice and aloe juice are effective remedies, and can be applied directly to a burn to relieve pain. Pumpkin pulp also has a soothing effect.

heatstroke

Kittens, old or overweight cats, and those with long coats, are most at risk. An affected cat will feel hot, will pant rapidly, will have dilated pupils and may collapse. Cool a victim rapidly: immerse the cat in cold water (hold the head above water) for at least 15 minutes or until the vet arrives. Hold an ice pack on the head and try to make the cat drink plenty of cold water, unless this causes vomiting.

aromatherapy

Mint may be massaged into the skin, especially in the head and neck area.

homoeopathy

Aconite and Glonoine (acute dosage) will alleviate early heatstroke.

Bach flowers

Rescue Remedy will reduce shock.

minor therapies

biochemical tissue salts

Nat. mur. and Ferr. phos. (acute dosage) should be given alternately.

Chinese medicine

Radish, bitter gourd (wild cucumber) and wax gourd (winter melon) are helpful if the cat is conscious: ½ tsp of these foods, well-chopped, should be offered.

skin

If there is one part of a cat's body that has the largest variety of persistent problems that fail to respond to conventional treatment, it is the skin and its attendant diseases. I see more referral cases for skin disorders than for all other problems put together, and I have treated cats who have been on medication for skin disease for over a decade. Natural medicines may not cure all cases, but their success rate is surprisingly high.

abscess

An abscess may be under the skin rather than within it, but it will be visible at the skin's surface. It may occur due to bacterial infection of a bite or wound, or following the penetration of a foreign body. You can apply a proprietary herbal drawing ointment, or a poultice of cabbage, turnip or parsnip, to bring the abscess to a 'head' and discharge the pus. Boil the vegetables until soft, strain, mash well, spread over a bandage and apply (the poultice should be warm, not hot). Keep it in place with layers of bandage. Alternatively, warm salty water will help to 'draw' an abscess.

Signs and symptoms An abscess is obvious as a painful swelling, which may discharge pus.

aromatherapy
Lavender and St John's wort will have a soothing effect, and should be massaged gently around the site of the abscess.

homoeopathy
Apis mel. is helpful for a hot, red, shiny abscess; Graphites for a cyst that becomes infected; Hepar sulph. for an active, discharging abscess; and Lachesis for a painful, purplish abscess (all in acute dosage). Silicea (chronic dosage) is another good remedy that will help to heal a longstanding abscess.

herbal medicine
Garlic and Echinacea will hasten the healing process.

Bach flowers
Rock rose is helpful for an abscess that is very painful to the touch.

minor therapies
biochemical tissue salts
Ferr. phos. will be beneficial if given in the early, acute stage; Silica may then be given while the abscess is discharging pus (both remedies in acute dosage). Calc. phos. (chronic dosage) will help subsequent healing of the skin.

Chinese medicine
Castor beans may be ground into a powder, and then applied directly to the abscess: this will help to promote rapid healing. Note: Castor beans must only be given externally – never administer the powder by mouth.

alopecia

There are no instant cures for hair loss, although natural remedies can help to promote hair growth on thinning or bald patches. Alopecia may result from a hormonal imbalance, a poor diet, a burn, allergies, immune-system disease, infections, parasites or ageing.

Signs and symptoms Hair loss may be generalized, or in patches. If the balding is bilaterally symmetrical (the same on either side), the cause is likely to be hormonal.

aromatherapy

Rosemary, and also Lavender with Calamus, with Terebinth and Pine, or with Thyme and Cedar, are all excellent and effective essential oils to massage into hairless areas of a cat's skin.

aromatherapy helps hair growth

Fred was one of those ordinary black cats with an ordinary name who live unexceptional lives, giving great joy to their owners. At 15 years of age, Fred was growing old gracefully and had never experienced a day's illness in his long life, but his coat was becoming noticeably thinner. His owner described him – quite accurately – as looking 'moth-eaten'.

A thorough clinical examination revealed no underlying health problems that might be causing the loss of hair: Fred was simply going bald as part of the process of ageing. His owner was interested in the use of natural therapies, and so I prescribed a course of massage with the essential oils of Rosemary and Thyme, to be carried out twice weekly.

Within a few weeks of this treatment we were rewarded by the appearance of a few new, wispy hairs on Fred's body. Over a period of several months, these gradually thickened into a reasonable covering of the bald areas and greatly improved his overall appearance.

homoeopathy

The following may be used (all in chronic dosage): Sepia alternating with Pulsatilla (in the case of female hormonal hair loss); Thallium as a general homoeopathic hair restorer; and Arsen. alb, for loss of the coat accompanied by itching and dandruff.

herbal medicine

Apple-cider vinegar may be added to drinking water at the rate of 5 ml (1 tsp) per 600 ml (1 pt), and Seaweed or Kelp powder added to the diet. Dandelion makes a good infusion. Burdock-root oil may be beneficial when massaged directly into the skin, especially if the skin is dry and scurfy (scaling). Nettle with Birch and Burdock may also be used for massage.

minor therapies

biochemical tissue salts

Kali. sulph. is helpful for bald areas with moist, sticky skin; Nat. mur. for bald areas with dry, scurfy skin; and silica for bald areas with a dull, non-glossy skin (all chronic dosage).

crystals and gems

Sapphire (liquid-gem remedy) may be given by mouth or added to water.

acute eczema

 There are almost innumerable possible causes for this condition (also commonly known as dermatitis). However, common causes include the presence of parasites, a bacterial or yeast infection, allergies, auto-immune skin diseases and injuries (including contact with chemicals). The following remedies are very helpful for 'wet' eczema and infected eczema (pyoderma).

Signs and symptoms Acute inflammation, soreness, redness and itching of the skin, causing excessive scratching or self-grooming.

aromatherapy

A combination of Rosemary and Lavender, or Terebinth, Lavender and Pine, may be massaged into the skin (but not directly into infected, wet or very inflamed areas).

homoeopathy

Hypericum with Calendula tincture may be diluted (three drops per 15 ml [3 tsps] of sterile water) and applied directly to the skin. The following (all acute dosage) may also provide relief: Apis mel. for allergic reactions and swollen, shiny skin; Cantharis for burning, painful skin eruptions; Hepar sulph. for infected skin (pyoderma); Psorinum for hot, smelly and very itchy skin (if the cat prefers the heat); and Sulphur for hot, itchy skin (if the cat lies in cool places).

herbal medicine

A decoction or infusion of Oak bark, or a decoction of Mallow, may be applied as a compress. Aloe vera gel, also applied directly, will soothe inflamed areas. Camomile may be given as an infusion by mouth.

Chinese medicine advises adding the foods shown here to a cat's daily diet, to alleviate the symptoms of eczema.

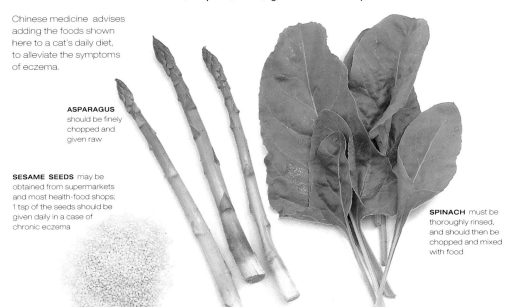

ASPARAGUS should be finely chopped and given raw

SESAME SEEDS may be obtained from supermarkets and most health-food shops; 1 tsp of the seeds should be given daily in a case of chronic eczema

SPINACH must be thoroughly rinsed, and should then be chopped and mixed with food

Bach flowers

Crabapple will improve dirty-looking, infected skin, and may also be helpful when an affected cat is depressed and miserable; Impatiens is beneficial for the hot, itchy skin of a nervous, excitable cat. As with all the Bach remedies, these may be given as drops by mouth or in the form of proprietary tablets.

minor therapies

biochemical tissue salts

Ferr. phos. (acute dosage) may help to relieve the symptoms.

Chinese medicine

Spinach, asparagus and crab (1 tsp of each, daily) may be given.

crystals and gems

Sapphire (liquid-gem remedy) may be given by mouth or added to water.

chronic eczema

The symptoms of this longstanding skin condition often respond well to the following natural medicines.

Signs and symptoms Persistent itchiness and soreness, often with hair loss. The skin usually stays dry, but may be greasy (seborrhoea).

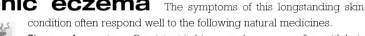

aromatherapy

A combination of Cedar, Thyme and Lavender, or of Rosemary and Lavender, may be used for massage to reduce the inflammation.

homoeopathy

The following may be given in chronic dosage: Acid. nit. for inflammation where the skin meets mucous membranes (such as at the lips and anus); Ant. crud. for scabs with a sticky secretion; Arsen. alb. for dry, flaky skin; Lycopodium for thickened skin with hair loss; Urtica for itchy, 'nettle-rash' symptoms; Nat. mur. for dry skin, especially at the bends of the limbs; and Pulex for flea allergies.

herbal medicine

Evening primrose oil is especially helpful when combined with Cod-liver oil. Nettle, Meadowsweet and

Dandelion may be given as infusions. Pine, Beech, Birch and Juniper may be used in the form of herbal tar on the skin (this tar is available only from herbalist shops and should be used under a herbalist's expert guidance, as it can be an irritant if wrongly used).

Bach flowers

Crabapple is a very effective 'cleansing' remedy.

minor therapies

biochemical tissue salts

Kali sulph. is beneficial for greasy skin; Nat. mur. for very dry skin (both in chronic dosage).

Chinese medicine

1 tsp of sesame seeds should be added to food daily.

crystals and gems

Liquid-remedy Sapphire may be given.

stud tail This is a condition mainly seen in unneutered male cats (although it occasionally occurs in females and in neutered males), in which glands beneath the skin in the area of the upper tail surface produce a greasy secretion. The cause of the condition is unknown, but it is probably the result of a hormonal imbalance. The homoeopathic remedy below will be helpful; stud tail should also be treated as for chronic eczema (see page 63), and for alopecia (see page 61) if bald patches appear in the affected area.

Signs and symptoms A yellow-brown, greasy secretion on the upper surface of the tail. The fur will also become matted, and bald patches may appear.

aromatherapy
Teatree-oil lotion should be used to clean the affected area twice daily; this is best applied with clean, soft cotton pads, which should be used once only before being discarded.

anal-gland disorders The anal glands are scent glands that are located on either side of the anus. They sometimes become blocked, which will lead to irritation, and sometimes become infected. The causes of these conditions are unknown, although an insufficient intake of fibre in the diet may predispose blockages (for advice on feeding a balanced diet, see pages 41–5). Blocked glands must be emptied by a vet.

Signs and symptoms Itchiness around the anus is a typical symptom, and an affected cat may rub his or her bottom on the ground, or suddenly look around as though feeling a shooting pain.

homoeopathy
Hepar sulph. (acute dosage) may be used if the glands are infected. Silicea (chronic dosage) is a good remedy for a cat who suffers from recurrent blockage of the anal glands.

herbal medicine
Garlic is often very helpful: ⅓ raw, chopped clove should be added to food daily. Alternatively, 2 mg Garlic oil daily, given as capsules, makes a good substitute for a cat who dislikes the taste of garlic.

minor therapies
biochemical tissue salts
Calc. phos. alternating with Nat. mur. (acute dosage) should be given in a case of acute inflammation and blockage of the anal glands. Silica (chronic dosage) will be beneficial for chronic, recurrent blockage of the glands.

warts

Warts are usually harmless, but can become infected. They may occur due to a viral infection, or simply as part of the ageing process.

Signs and symptoms Warts may range in shape from 'cauliflower-like' to sessile (flat).

homoeopathy

Thuja tincture should be applied as one drop on each wart daily. Causticum (chronic dosage) may be a beneficial remedy for an old, stiff, warty cat.

herbal medicine

Greater-celandine juice may be applied to a wart daily. Alternatively, slices of fresh Garlic or Banana skin (see right) may be applied to cover the wart and surrounding area. Milk thistle may be helpful when given as an infusion.

minor therapies

biochemical tissue salts

Kali mur. may be given alternately with Nat. mur. (both remedies in chronic dosage).

Chinese medicine

Peanuts and brown sugar should be ground together and given in the form of an infusion.

crystals and gems

Coral may be an effective remedy for a cat who is prone to developing warts. It should be placed next to the cat when he or she is at rest, as close as possible to the area of the wart or warts, for up to two hours a day. Alternatively, liquid-remedy Coral may be given by mouth or added to drinking water.

covering a wart

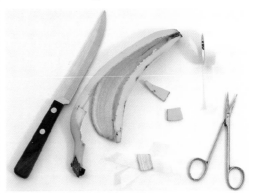

1 Banana skin is a very good remedy for warts, and often produces rapid results. Cut a square of freshly peeled Banana skin, large enough to cover the entire area of the wart.

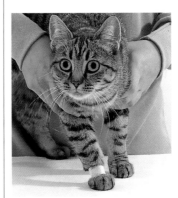

2 Place the Banana skin over the wart, and secure it with medical adhesive tape (take great care that this is not too tight). Replace daily.

ears and eyes

Cats may begin to lose their acute sense of hearing or to suffer from failing eyesight as part of the ageing process, but those kept indoors generally cope well with this gradual change and increasingly find their way about by smell. Ears and eyes are complicated organs, and any disease should be treated as soon as possible. In younger cats, ear problems can occur in three areas: the ear flap, the ear canal, and the middle and inner ear. A cat's eye is also extremely complex and has many components, of which the eyelids, conjunctiva, cornea, lens, iris and retina are the main structures. Some of the most common conditions to affect the ears and eyes are included in this section.

otitis externa

Otitis externa is a general term used to describe inflammation of the ear canal. This may be due to the presence of ear mites (see page 116); to a foreign body such as a grass awn, polyp or tumour; or to a bacterial, fungal or yeast infection.

Signs and symptoms Excessive head-shaking and ear-scratching. There may be a visible discharge and an unpleasant odour emanating from the ear canal.

aromatherapy

Clove and Thyme may be massaged into the skin near the ears to soothe the inflammation. A good general cleansing agent can be made from 2.5 ml (½ tsp) of warm Olive oil with a few drops of Lemon juice: this may be used to clean the outer part of the ear. A few drops should be allowed to drain into the ear canal, and the ear then gently massaged at its base. This will soothe the irritation and encourage any excess wax or discharge to come out. Do not attempt to clean inside the ear canal, and never use cotton buds: the tissues are easily damaged, and any wax that is on its way out could be pushed back and impacted.

homoeopathy

Hypericum with Calendula lotion is a good homoeopathic cleansing agent. For internal use, the following may

Calc. sulph. clears ears

Purdy was a four-year-old British blue who, since kittenhood, had suffered from chronic otitis externa. Antibiotics, steroids and cleaning of the ears under anaesthetic had all failed to prevent the constant recurrence of a blood-stained, purulent discharge from both ears.

Persistent ear discharges are notoriously hard to resolve, and I explained to Purdy's owner that, although natural medicines might well be very helpful, they were unlikely to clear the problem entirely. However, Purdy began a twice-daily dose of the biochemical tissue salt Calc. sulph. Three weeks later, her ears were clean and dry, with no smell and no discharge.

help (acute dosage in a severe case, chronic dosage in a longstanding one): Graphites for a sticky, smelly discharge; Hepar sulph. for an infected, purulent discharge; and Psorinum for a hot, itchy ear (if the cat prefers to be warm) or sulphur (if the cat prefers to be cool).

herbal medicine

A very good herbal cleansing agent comprises three parts Rosemary infusion mixed with one part Witch-hazel lotion. An effective cleansing remedy when ear mites are present (see page 116) is made of equal parts of Thyme, Rosemary and Rue infusions, mixed 50:50 with Olive oil. An infusion of Thyme will soothe the inflammation and reduce irritation.

minor therapies
biochemical tissue salts

The following are all helpful. Acute dosage should be administered for a severe case, chronic dosage for a longstanding problem: Calc. sulph. for a profuse discharge that also contains blood; Ferr. phos. for a hot, painful ear; or Kali sulph. for a yellow, catarrhal discharge.

crystals and gems

Sapphire (liquid-gem remedy) may be given by mouth or added to water.

haematoma

This is a haemorrhage that occurs within the ear flap, causing it to swell. The causes of this condition include trauma (for example, from banging the ear against a hard object, or trapping the ear in a door), the presence of parasites in the ear canal, and infection in the ear canal. Surgery to drain the haematoma followed by suturing of the ear flap to prevent further haemorrhaging is usually advised, although haematomas do have a tendency to recur, making repeat surgery necessary. However, surgery can often be avoided altogether by using natural medicines.

Signs and symptoms Violent head-shaking or head-rubbing, and a swollen ear flap.

homoeopathy

Arnica given in acute dosage for three days, followed by Hamamelis in chronic dosage for two weeks, may reduce the swelling.

herbal medicine

Witch-hazel lotion may be applied directly to the ear flap. Clean, soft cotton pads should be used for this, with each pad used only once and then discarded.

minor therapies
biochemical tissue salts

Ferr. phos. (acute dosage) may help to reduce the swelling and allow the blood to clot and be re-absorbed.

otitis media and otitis interna

Most middle- and inner-ear problems are caused by an inward spread of otitis externa (see pages 66–7). Infection can also travel from the throat via the Eustachian tube The causes of otitis media and interna include bacterial and fungal infections, and (occasionally) tumours.

Signs and symptoms Head-shaking and ear-scratching; an affected cat may also tilt his or her head to one side and show an obvious loss of balance (for example, inability to walk in a straight line).

aromatherapy
Rosemary and Thyme may be gently massaged near the ear in order to relieve irritation.

homoeopathy
Hepar sulph. (acute dosage) is ideal for symptoms that have developed only recently; Merc. cor. (chronic dosage) is recommended for a longstanding problem.

Bach flowers
Scleranthus can be helpful if the condition is affecting a cat's balance.

minor therapies
biochemical tissue salts
Kali mur. (acute dosage) may be given to relieve the symptoms.
crystals and gems
Sapphire (liquid-gem remedy) may be given by mouth or added to water.

conjunctivitis

Conjunctivitis is an inflammation of the pink mucous membrane surrounding the 'white' of the eye. It is a common problem in cats. The condition may be caused by a viral or bacterial infection (see chlamydia on page 119), a foreign body, an allergy, entropion (eyelids or eyelashes rubbing the eye) or physical trauma.

Signs and symptoms Red, sore-looking eyes with accompanying discharge. The cat may paw at the eyes or rub his or her face along the ground in an attempt to relieve irritation.

homoeopathy
The following may be used (in acute dosage): Apis mel. for sore eyes with swollen eyelids and/or conjunctiva; Arsen. alb. for watery, inflamed eyes with a thin, acrid discharge; Kali bich. for a thick, green, stringy discharge; and Pulsatilla for a creamy, catarrhal discharge with little discomfort.

herbal medicine
Greater-celandine or Dock infusion may be used to bathe the eyes three times daily. A fresh infusion should be made up each day, and kept cool and covered when not in use. Eyebright may be used in the same way, or given orally, as can an infusion or diluted tincture of Goldenseal.

minor therapies

biochemical tissue salts

The following are suitable remedies for conjunctivitis (all in acute dosage): Ferr. phos. when no discharge is present; Kali mur. for a white discharge; Nat. phos. for a sticky yellow discharge; and Silica where styes (small, reddened swellings on the eyelid) are evident.

Chinese medicine

Cucumber juice – freshly squeezed on each occasion – may be applied directly (one drop in each eye, three times daily). Alternatively, ½ tsp of diced water chestnut may be added to food twice daily.

crystals and gems

Pearl (liquid-gem remedy) may be given by mouth or added to water.

administering eye drops

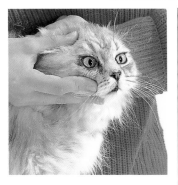

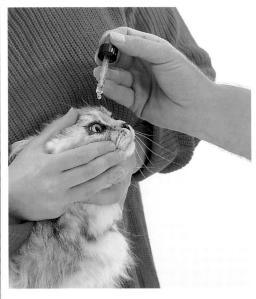

1 Small bottles with droppers in the lids are available from pharmacies. If you wish to re-use a bottle that you already have, be sure to clean it very thoroughly with hot water, and then leave it to air-dry, before use. Giving eye drops will be easier if you have the help of an assistant to restrain the cat properly; alternatively, position the cat against a solid surface so that he or she is not able to back away from you. Draw up the medicine into the dropper. Hold the cat's head with the fingers of one hand on either side of the affected eye, so that you can keep the eyelids apart.

2 Taking great care not to hold the dropper too close to the eyeball, in case the cat should make a sudden movement, carefully administer the drop or drops. Still holding the head, release the eyelids and allow the cat to blink several times: this will help to disperse the drops over the entire surface of the eyeball.

corneal ulceration

The cornea is the central, transparent area of the eye. It is very delicate – even tiny scratches may ulcerate rapidly – and, as it has no direct blood supply, it heals slowly. As well as resulting from injury, a corneal ulcer may be caused by infection or the presence of a foreign body, by entropion (rubbing eyelids or eyelashes), or by a deficiency in tear production.

Signs and symptoms The eye will be red, sore and discharging. The cat may rub his or her eye or face along the ground, and be photophobic (avoid bright light).

homoeopathy

The following remedies will be helpful: Argent. nit. (acute dosage) for a painful eye, with accompanying redness and soreness; Merc. cor. for pain and photophobia (the cat may also be thirsty); and Silicea (chronic dosage), to help to heal the scarring resulting from an old ulcer.

herbal medicine

An infusion of Greater celandine may be applied directly to the eye to help to relieve symptoms of redness and irritation. An infusion or tincture (the tincture to be diluted by adding three drops to 10 ml [2 tsps] sterile water) of Eyebright or Goldenseal may also be used in this way, or given orally.

epiphora

This condition involves an overflow of tears. It often results from another eye condition such as conjunctivitis (see pages 68–9) or corneal ulceration (see above), although – even in the absence of disease – some cats' eyes permanently discharge. Where no other eye disease is present, the usual cause of epiphora is deficient drainage of tears through the nasolacrimal (tear) duct.

Signs and symptoms Dark tear staining on the cat's face, running from the inner corners of the eyes down the muzzle. Strangely, white cats seem to be most prone to epiphora, which makes the staining even more obvious!

homoeopathy

Allium cepa (chronic dosage) should be administered.

herbal medicine

A diluted tincture or infusion of Eyebright may be used to bathe the eyes twice daily. A fresh solution should be made up each day, and always kept cool and covered between applications.

minor therapies
biochemical tissue salts

Nat. mur. (chronic dosage) is a good remedy for persistent epiphora.

cataract

This is an opacity of the lens – the part of the eye that focuses the light passing through it on to the retina. For light to travel through the lens, it must be transparent. Any opacity will therefore cause defective vision and, if the cataract progresses, blindness. A cataract or cataracts can be congenital, or may develop with age. Poisoning, diabetes mellitus (see pages 82–3) and infection can also cause them.

Signs and symptoms Obvious visual impairment, and a blue or white opacity of the lens.

homoeopathy
Cineraria eye lotion should be used twice daily. The following are also helpful: Calc. carb. for an overweight, old cat; Conium mac. for an old, weak cat, especially with weakened hindquarters; and Phosphorus for a thin, older cat (all chronic dosage).

herbal medicine
An infusion of Greater celandine may be beneficial.

minor therapies
biochemical tissue salts
Nat. mur. is a good remedy for recent cataracts; Silica is suitable for established cataracts (both to be given in chronic dosage).

supplements
Supplement the diet with Vitamin E (100 iu daily) and Selenium (25 mg daily) to help slow down cataract development. Natural Vitamin E should be used (see page 47).

glaucoma
Glaucoma is an increase of pressure inside the eyeball. The eyeball is filled with a fluid that is constantly secreted and drained, but, if anything disturbs this balance, pressure builds up with a rapid risk of causing permanent damage and blindness. The condition may occur because of congenital abnormalities in drainage, or may be the result of infection, inflammation or a tumour.

Signs and symptoms The affected eye will be extremely painful and may be swollen.

homoeopathy
Belladonna or Phosphorus (both in acute dosage) may be given to relieve discomfort and swelling. Euphrasia tincture, applied after dilution (three drops in 10 ml [2 tsps] sterile water) using an eyebath, will help to soothe and cleanse the eye.

minor therapies
supplements
Cod-liver oil is a very good source of Vitamins A and D, both of which will help to accelerate the healing process. Three drops of oil should be given three times daily with food, for up to 10 days.

respiratory system

Unlike dogs, cats are exceedingly prone to problems affecting the upper respiratory tract, such as sneezing, colds and flu. The lifestyle of an individual will also be a factor: a cat who lives permanently indoors will obviously be less at risk than one who regularly encounters many other cats.

One of the most common respiratory disorders that I see in cats brought in for treatment with natural therapy is in the unfortunate individuals who were affected by a bout of feline viral upper-respiratory-tract disease – more commonly known as cat 'flu (see page 118) – at an early age and, several years on, are still experiencing persistent coughing, sneezing, nasal discharge and sinusitis.

In these types of cases, antibiotics never seem to clear the symptoms for long, but natural medicines can often be extremely helpful.

sneezing, nasal discharge
and sinusitis

The upper part of the respiratory tract is a common site for disease symptoms. An acute infection can cause serious illness, while sinusitis can be chronic and debilitating. Causes may be infection (either bacterial or viral, especially the cat 'flu virus), or the presence of a foreign body (such as a grass awn) or tumours.

Signs and symptoms Sneezing, head-shaking, and a purulent discharge from one or both nostrils. A cat may stop eating if the nostrils or sinuses are blocked.

aromatherapy

Eucalyptus, Hyssop, Myrrh, Pine, Teatree, Terebinth and Thyme may all be given by diffusion or massage.

homoeopathy

The following will be helpful (all in chronic dosage): Kali bich. for a yellow, tough, stringy discharge; Pulsatilla for a bland, catarrhal, profuse discharge; and Silicea for chronic, intractable sinusitis.

herbal medicine

Infusions of Goldenseal, Garlic or Liquorice will be beneficial.

minor therapies

biochemical tissue salts

The following may all be given: Ferr. phos. (acute dosage) for severe sinusitis; Kali mur. (chronic dosage) when catarrhal, white mucus is present; Kali sulph. (chronic dosage) when yellow, thick mucus is present; and Nat. mur. (chronic dosage) for a watery, thin discharge.

Chinese medicine

1 tsp of cornsilk or onion leaf may be given, chopped, daily.

crystals and gems

Pearl (liquid-gem remedy) may be given by mouth or added to water.

coughing

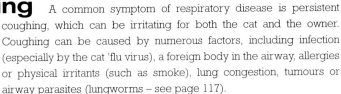

A common symptom of respiratory disease is persistent coughing, which can be irritating for both the cat and the owner. Coughing can be caused by numerous factors, including infection (especially by the cat 'flu virus), a foreign body in the airway, allergies or physical irritants (such as smoke), lung congestion, tumours or airway parasites (lungworms – see page 117).

Signs and symptoms The frequent bouts of coughing may be productive (accompanied by mucus) or non-productive (dry).

aromatherapy

Eucalyptus, Hyssop, Myrrh, Pine, Teatree, Terebinth and Thyme may all be given by diffusion or massage.

homoeopathy

The following will help (all given in chronic dosage): Arsen. alb. for harsh coughing that is worse at night; Bryonia for a dry, hacking cough that is worse in the morning; Ipecac. syrup for spasmodic coughing with vomiting; Spongia for coughing linked to a heart problem; Rumex crispus for coughing that improves at night; and Drosera for a sensitive larynx.

herbal medicine

Sage, Thyme, Ribwort plantain, Coltsfoot and Liquorice may be given as infusions. Mullein is soothing for coughing that is worse at night.

minor therapies

biochemical tissue salts

Ferr. phos. (acute dosage) should be given for an acute, dry, hard cough. The following will also help (all in chronic dosage): Calc. sulph. for a loose, rattling cough; Kali mur. for coughing with white mucus; Kali sulph. for yellow mucus; Mag. phos. for spasmodic, persistent coughing; and Silica for coughing with a profuse, yellow-green mucus.

Chinese medicine

Ginger, spearmint and grapes should be given (1 tsp daily). Lemon is ideal for coughing accompanied by mucus; strawberries for a dry cough; and pumpkin for bronchial asthma.

strawberries cure coughing

Molly suffered from a persistent dry cough, which no amount of treatment – conventional or natural – had been able to clear.

While adding to my already copious notes on Molly, I asked her owner more about her eating habits, and discovered that she liked strawberries: a fairly unusual taste among cats. While trying another homoeopathic remedy, I also suggested that, as in Chinese food medicine strawberries can relieve dry coughs, Molly should be given the treat of a strawberry each day. Whether it was the homoeopathic remedy or the strawberries I shall never be entirely sure, but there is no doubting the fact that Molly no longer coughs. To be on the safe side – and because she loves them – her owner still gives her the daily strawberry.

asthma

Asthma in cats – as in humans – is an allergic condition that is always difficult to treat using conventional methods.

Signs and symptoms Wheezing and difficulty in breathing, coughing and a congested chest.

aromatherapy

Eucalyptus, given by massage or via a diffuser, will help to clear the airways.

homoeopathy

The following remedies are useful (all in chronic dosage): Bryonia for asthma that is accompanied by a dry cough, which worsens when the cat moves about; Drosera for a sensitive throat and a spasmodic, dry cough; Rumex crispus for asthma with a frothy mucus discharge from the nose and throat; and Sulphur for chesty asthma that worsens in warm conditions.

herbal medicine

Garlic is a good remedy for asthma: ⅓ raw, chopped clove should be added to the food daily. Alternatively, if the cat refuses to eat food that has been 'doctored' with Garlic, 2 mg Garlic oil, in the form of capsules, may be given daily.

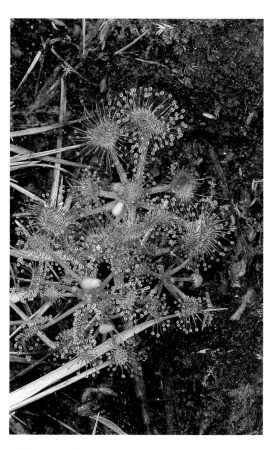

minor therapies

biochemical tissue salts

The following should all be given in chronic dosage: Kali phos. for asthma resembling human hay fever; Calc. phos. for bronchial asthma that is accompanied by a thick, clear mucus; and Kali sulph. for bronchial asthma with yellow mucus.

Chinese medicine

Root ginger (¼ tsp, grated) or lychees (1 tsp of steamed, dried fruit) may be added to food daily.

crystals and gems

Pearl (liquid-gem remedy) may be given directly by mouth or added to drinking water.

As well as being one of the few insect-eating plants, Sundew (Drosera) is often used by homoeopaths as a remedy for tickly coughs.

pneumonia

Pneumonia is as serious a problem in cats as it is in humans. The causes of the condition are infection (especially viral, but it can also be bacterial and fungal), or the presence of a foreign body or tumour.

Signs and symptoms Coughing, rapid breathing, fever and chest pain.

aromatherapy
Eucalyptus, Hyssop, Myrrh, Pine, Teatree, Terebinth and Thyme may be given by massage or diffusion.

homoeopathy
Aconite should be given at the first signs; Belladonna at the height of fever; Bryonia if the cat will not move; Phosphorus for coughed-up blood; and Sulphur for coughed-up yellow mucus (all in acute dosage).

herbal medicine
Garlic, Fenugreek and Nasturtium leaves are all effective remedies.

minor therapies
biochemical tissue salts
Ferr. phos. (acute dosage) is suitable for a case of acute pneumonia; Kali mur. (acute dosage) for pneumonia with congested lungs and the production of a thick mucus; and Silica (chronic dosage) for persistent pneumonia and scarred lungs.
Chinese medicine
Saffron, grapefruit peel, tangerine or beetroot (1 tsp) may be given while pneumonia is acute.
crystals and gems
Pearl (liquid-gem remedy) may be given by mouth or added to water.

epistaxis

Epistaxis – otherwise known as a nose bleed – is alarming when in full flow, but it can often be arrested with natural medicines. A nose bleed is frequently caused by injury, or infection (especially the cat 'flu virus). It may also result from a tumour or a foreign body in the nasal passage.

Signs and symptoms Bleeding from one or both nostrils.

homoeopathy
Arnica (acute dosage) may be given at the start of bleeding, especially if the epistaxis is due to injury. Also useful (all in acute dosage) are Ipecac. for a nose bleed of bright red blood, with vomiting; Phosphorus for very persistent bleeding; and Melilotus for profuse bleeding.

minor therapies
biochemical tissue salts
Crush six Ferr. phos. tablets and apply them directly to the nostrils.
Chinese medicine
Water chestnuts, chives or vinegar may be given while the tendency to bleeding persists (no more than 5 ml [1 tsp] vinegar daily).

cardiovascular system

The diseases in this section cover the heart and the circulatory system of blood and lymph. As cats, on the whole, have a healthier lifestyle than humans (few cats drink alcohol or smoke!), heart disease and circulation problems are less commonly seen by vets than by doctors. However, cats can be slothful and so the early signs of heart disease – such as unusual tiredness, for example – can be missed. Natural medicines can be very effective for the cardiovascular conditions that do occur.

congestion

Many problems of the heart and circulatory system cause a build-up of fluid. This congestion, or oedema, may be evident as swollen feet or legs, or as fluid on the lungs or in the abdomen (known as ascites, or dropsy). A failing heart is a common cause of congestion, as the heart is unable to maintain the circulation of blood and excess fluid begins to pool in the tissues. Liver disease and tumours can contribute to oedema, and ascites is often a feature of feline infectious peritonitis (see page 118).

Signs and symptoms Swollen, puffy limbs in particular, or swelling in any part of the body; an enlarged, tense abdomen; weight loss; and lack of energy.

aromatherapy
Lemon, Birch, Sandalwood and Juniper may all be given by massage.

homoeopathy
The following should all be given in chronic dosage: Apis mel. for oedema where the skin remains 'pitted' after being pressed, and where the cat is not especially thirsty; Acetic acid and Eel serum for congestion (especially ascites) where the cat is quite thirsty; and Adonis and Digitalis for congestion with major heart disease.

herbal medicine
Bearberry, Dandelion, Dill seed, Ground elder, Hawthorn, Juniper berry, Parsley and Sloe berry, given by infusion, are all ideal for congested circulation. (Any of these remedies will be helpful if given on their own, and no more than two should be used at the same time.)

minor therapies
biochemical tissue salts
Calc. sulph. and Nat. sulph. are effective (both in chronic dosage); the latter is especially useful where there is liver disease.

Chinese medicine
Plums, broad-bean pods and mung beans are all recommended in Chinese medicine for use in a case of congestion, to be given as follows:

one diced plum on alternate days;
½ broad-bean pod, finely chopped,
daily; and ½ tsp of sprouted mung
beans daily.

crystals and gems
Liquid-remedy Pearl may be given.

supplements
If diuretics are being given (to
remove excess water), a Potassium
supplement may be necessary, as
diuretics cause an excessive loss of
Potassium (your vet will advise you).

heart disease
 Cats are sometimes born with heart defects, and they may also experience problems with the electrical control mechanisms of the heart. A common problem is congestive heart failure, where the heart cannot maintain a sufficient blood supply to body tissues. The following natural medicines are all compatible with any prescribed drugs. It is also sensible to reduce the intake of salt in food, to encourage weight loss in an obese cat (see page 45), and to promote gentle exercise.

Signs and symptoms Breathlessness, coughing, unwillingness to exercise, oedema and ascites (see opposite), weight loss and liver disease (see page 99).

aromatherapy
Mint given by massage will help heart
and circulatory problems.

homoeopathy
The following are helpful (all in
chronic dosage): Crataegus and
Digitalis for a weak heart and poor
circulation; Spongia tosta and Rumex
crispus for associated coughing;
cactus grand. for pain; Lycopus if the
heartbeat is rapid; and Adonis and
Strophanthus for valve problems.
Laurocerasus is beneficial where the
lungs are congested and there is
cyanosis (poor oxygenation of the
blood); the tincture may also be
given (one drop every 15 minutes
for up to two hours) where there
is a danger of cyanosis.

herbal medicine
Capsicum, Rosemary and Convallaria
are all suitable: infusions of one or
more of these will encourage the
removal of excess fluid and promote
a more efficient heart function.

minor therapies
biochemical tissue salts
Calc. fluor. (chronic dosage) will
improve the strength of the heart
muscle; Kali phos. (also in chronic
dosage) will act to stabilize electric
abnormalities in the heart.
Chinese medicine
Sweetcorn and wholewheat should
be given (½ tsp).
crystals and gems
Ruby (liquid-gem remedy) may be
given by mouth or added to water.

anaemia

Anaemia is a lack of red blood cells. Blood loss through haemorrhaging after an accident, or following the ingestion of certain poisons such as warfarin (or mouse and rat poison – this stops the blood from clotting), may cause anaemia. Other poisons (for example, heavy metals, such as lead) will have the same effect by destroying the body's red blood cells. A heavy parasite infestation, feline infectious anaemia (see page 118) and diseased organs (as in kidney failure) can also lead to anaemia.

Signs and symptoms Pale lips and gums, and general weakness.

aromatherapy

Marjoram given by massage will help to rejuvenate a weak, anaemic cat.

using combined remedies

Unfortunately, Samson was a good mouser. He caught and dispatched mice regularly, always eating them but leaving the tails behind (usually behind the sofa, where they would be found some days later).

I use the word unfortunately, because on one occasion Samson's proficiency was his undoing: he ate a mouse which had just swallowed a dose of mouse poison. Samson began to bleed internally, as the poison in question kills by preventing the blood from clotting normally, so that haemorrhaging occurs. Despite the antidote (Vitamin K) being given, Samson was still extremely anaemic.

I decided to attack the problem using a mixture of homoeopathy (Crotalus horridus), herbs (Blackberries and Parsley), Bach flower essence (Hornbeam) and biochemical tissue salts (Ferr. phos.). The intensive treatment soon had Samson back to threaten the mouse population once again, and also demonstrates how – in such a situation – a variety of natural medicines can be used to accelerate healing.

homoeopathy

The following should all be given in chronic dosage: China officinalis for debility; Crotalus horridus for warfarin poisoning; Ferrum met. where poor nutrition is a factor; Cuprum met. where insufficient red blood cells are produced; Lachesis if the disease causes dark haemorrhages; Lycopodium for excessive destruction of red blood cells; Phosphorus where persistent bleeding of bright red blood is contributing to the anaemia; Secale for haemorrhages under the skin; and Acid. phos. to reduce weakness, especially in a young cat.

herbal medicine

Nettles and Parsley are beneficial, either as infusions or chopped and added to food. Black-berry fruits – Bramble, Bilberry, Elderberry and Black grapes – are also useful singly or combined, and may be given as infusions or dietary supplements.

Bach flowers

Hornbeam is a strengthening remedy for the weary and weak.

minor therapies
biochemical tissue salts
Calc. phos., Nat. mur. and Ferr.
phos. (all in chronic dosage) help to
increase red-blood-cell production
and raise energy levels.

Chinese medicine
Dates, mung beans, spinach and
shiitake mushrooms are the food
remedies recommended in Chinese
medicine for anaemia. Where they
are available, the following should
be added to the affected cat's food:
1 tsp of chopped dates on alternate
days; ½ tsp of sprouted mung beans
daily; one chopped raw spinach leaf
daily; and ½ tsp of chopped shiitake
mushrooms daily.

crystals and gems
Ruby (liquid-gem remedy) may be
given by mouth or added to water.

supplements
Food and supplements rich in iron
and B-complex vitamins are especially
beneficial. Liver, Brewer's yeast, kelp,
royal jelly and green vegetables are
ideal. Extra Vitamin C can also be
of some help.

aortic thrombosis

This life-threatening condition occurs
when a blood clot forms where the aorta (the main blood vessel from
the heart) divides into two to supply the hindlegs. The cause is usually
an underlying heart problem. This condition needs urgent veterinary
attention, but natural medicines can be given immediately to
counteract collapse and shock.

Signs and symptoms The sudden onset of hindleg paralysis: the cat
may cry out in pain and will be in shock, and the hindlegs will rapidly
start to become cold.

homoeopathy
Aconite (acute dosage) is ideal for
this condition, and can be powdered
into the mouth. Carbo vegetabilis
and Ver. alb. (acute dosage) may
also be given.

herbal medicine
An infusion of Elder blossom will
help to allay shock.

Bach flowers
Rescue Remedy is – as in many
emergency situations – the ideal
remedy for a cat who is suffering
from shock and in pain; single drops
should be administered directly into
the mouth.

minor therapies
biochemical tissue salts
Nat. sulph. (acute dosage) can be
powdered into the cat's mouth to
alleviate shock.

crystals and gems
Pearl (liquid-gem remedy) may be
administered to the cat by mouth
in single drops.

lymph-gland disease

The lymphatic system is the body's drainage system, and the lymph glands act as detoxifying points along the route. Although linked with the circulation in general, the lymphatic system has its own set of diseases: lymphosarcoma, or cancer of the lymph glands, is one of these (see also pages 112–13). In addition, the lymph glands can become enlarged due to bacterial, viral or parasitic infection (see also toxoplasmosis on page 119), or due to immune-based arthritis (see pages 84–5).

Signs and symptoms One or more lymph glands become enlarged and hardened, and the cat will show signs of a general malaise (including a lack of energy and reluctance to eat). Enlarged glands under the chin, in front of the shoulder blades or behind the knees are normally fairly easy to feel.

homoeopathy

The following should be given (all in chronic dosage): Baryta carb. for lymph-gland enlargement in kittens and old cats; Calc. fluor. for very hard lymph glands; and Conium mac. for hardened glands in a weak cat, who may have urinary incontinence and weak hindlegs. Phytolacca in its homoeopathic form is particularly effective for enlarged throat glands, and for inflamed mammary lymph glands in a female cat.

herbal medicine

Echinacea or Phytolacca may be given by infusion. Seaweed shredded in apple cider can be applied locally to enlarged lymph glands, especially if the glands are hot and painful.

minor therapies

crystals and gems

Topaz (liquid-gem remedy) is useful: this may be given by mouth or added to drinking water.

homoeopathy relieves soreness

Johnson was a ginger tom who preferred to keep himself to himself, and spent most of his day asleep or eating. This peaceful existence was disturbed only by a recurrent sore throat. His owner was convinced that this was because Johnson's throat was the only part of him that he ever used to excess – either to swallow food, or to demand more.

Be that as it may, the sore throat was a problem, particularly because of the enlarged lymph glands that often persisted long after the actual soreness had subsided. Homoeopathic Phytolacca, given as one tablet three times daily for a week, followed by one tablet twice daily for three weeks, brought the glands down to their normal size.

Along with the judicious use of other homoeopathic remedies for sore throats, and further dosing with Phytolacca when the glands became enlarged, Johnson was finally freed from the only problem in his life, and now happily spends his days eating. Or asleep and presumably dreaming of eating.

endocrine system

This is the network of glands that produces the hormones that control body processes and metabolism. The most important glands in this system are the adrenal, thyroid and pituitary glands, and the areas of the pancreas that produce insulin (the Islets of Langerhans). Diseases of these glands are very difficult to control or to cure, and often need lifelong treatment: diabetes mellitus (see pages 82–3) is a well-known example. Although natural medicines may not be adequate on their own to effect cures or to control glandular problems, they are often an invaluable part of any treatment. With dedicated care from his or her owner, a diabetic cat, for example, may go on to have a long and happy life.

hyperthyroidism

The thyroid glands control a cat's body metabolism. Hyperthyroidism, an over-activity of the thyroid glands, causes a speeding-up of the metabolism; this results in a variety of symptoms, as many body processes are affected. The condition may be caused by cancer (see pages 112–13) or hyperplasia (a non-cancerous size increase of the thyroid glands). Conventional treatment usually involves giving drugs to relieve symptoms, or removing the glands surgically, but natural medicines can make this unnecessary.

Signs and symptoms Enlarged thyroid glands, restlessness, weight loss, increased heart and breathing rates, increased thirst and appetite, and weakness.

aromatherapy
Massage with Lavender, Melissa (Lemon balm) or Sweet marjoram will help to calm a hyperthyroid cat: this is very beneficial, as restlessness is a key symptom of the condition.

homoeopathy
Nat. mur. (chronic dosage) will help to alleviate heightened thirst, and will also curtail further loss of weight and increased weakness.

herbal medicine
Bugle weed and Motherwort may be given as infusions.

Bach flowers
Impatiens reduces the irritability and unsettled nature of an affected cat.

minor therapies
biochemical tissue salts
Kali phos. (chronic dosage) calms the restlessness yet weakness that is characteristic of hyperthyroidism.
Chinese medicine
Logan fruit reduces restlessness, palpitations and weight loss; one fruit should be given every three days.
crystals and gems
Liquid-remedy Pearl may be given by mouth or added to drinking water.

diabetes mellitus
This condition results from a deficiency of the hormone insulin, which is needed to transfer glucose from the blood into body tissues: it causes the body to become 'starved' of glucose. Diabetes can be caused by pancreatic disease and damage, by misuse of drugs such as steroids and hormones, and by obesity (see page 45). Regular injections of insulin may be required, but natural medicines can reduce the need for them.

Signs and symptoms Excessive thirst and hunger, lethargy and cataracts (see page 71).

aromatherapy
Eucalyptus, Juniper and Lemon may be used for massage.

homoeopathy
Syzygium and Iris vers. should be given in chronic dosage (continued dosage may vary: consult your vet).

herbal medicine
Oak bark, Olive root and Haricot-bean pods may all be used to make decoctions. Regular administration of one or more of these remedies may help to reduce the quantity of insulin required (although they are unlikely to remove the need for it altogether).

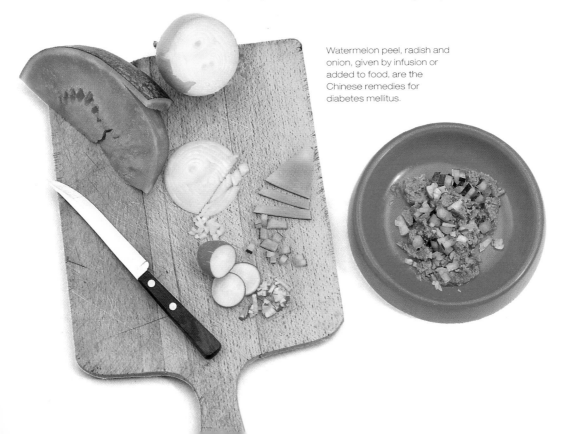

Watermelon peel, radish and onion, given by infusion or added to food, are the Chinese remedies for diabetes mellitus.

Bach flowers
Hornbeam and Olive can help to reduce the lethargy and weakness caused by diabetes.

minor therapies
biochemical tissue salts
Nat. mur. and Nat. sulph. should be administered alternately (both in chronic dosage).
Chinese medicine
Ginseng may be administered as proprietary tablets (50 mg daily), or as ¼ tsp of the diced root daily. Watermelon peel, radish and onion may also be given in the form of a daily infusion.
crystals and gems
Diamond (liquid-gem remedy) may be given by mouth or added to water.

eliminating the need for insulin
Ernest was a Persian, recently diagnosed with diabetes mellitus. His owner wished to avoid insulin injections, and so came to me. Ernest was only mildly diabetic, was in good general condition and had no other health problems.

I instigated acupuncture and homoeopathy treatment. The acupuncture sessions took place weekly for four weeks, then every two weeks, then at four-weekly intervals. Syzygium was the homoeopathic remedy used, given three times daily for one week, twice daily for four weeks, once daily for four weeks, then twice weekly.

In the first eight weeks Ernest was perfectly well, but lost weight. However, this then rose again and stabilized. Blood tests still show a very mild diabetes, but it seems to be held in check by the treatment, with no need for insulin.

hypokalaemia

Hypokalaemia is a deficiency of potassium in the blood, and is a condition seen mainly in older cats. Kidney disease (see page 104) can result in excess potassium excretion from the body, as can persistent diarrhoea (see page 101). A dietary deficiency can also occur, especially in a chronically ill cat. As well as using the following natural medicines, any underlying cause will need to be treated.

Signs and symptoms General muscle weakness: this can lead to breathing difficulty, weight loss, poor coat condition and anaemia (see pages 78–9).

homoeopathy
Kali chlor. (to be administered in chronic dosage) is a suitable remedy if the hypokalaemia has been caused by the onset of kidney disease (see page 104). Kali carb. (also to be given in chronic dosage) is ideal for a weakened, older cat.

minor therapies
biochemical tissue salts
Kali sulph. should be alternated with Kali phos. (both in chronic dosage).
crystals and gems
Liquid-remedy Ruby may be given.
supplements
Potassium is a useful supplement.

musculo-skeletal system

This body system consists of the muscles, bones, joints, tendons and ligaments, which give the body shape and enable it to move. They are the parts that tend to suffer most from mechanical wear and tear, injury and inflammation, and can be very difficult to put right once they have gone wrong. Of the natural therapies that are available, acupuncture and T-touch massage (see pages 30–1) can be beneficial for any disorder of the musculo-skeletal system; osteopathy and chiropractic (see page 36) are also extremely helpful in many cases.

osteoarthritis

Arthritis, or inflammation of one or more joints (especially the shoulder and elbow) is mainly a problem of the older cat. Osteoarthritis is caused by the wear and tear of old age, but joint inflammation in younger cats does occur occasionally, due to injury to the bones, infection or disease of the immune system.

Signs and symptoms Stiffness, and pain in the arthritic joints which causes lameness.

aromatherapy

Juniper, Birch, Pine, Thyme, Terebinth and Rosemary are all appropriate remedies to use for massage.

homoeopathy

The following can all be given (in chronic dosage, unless stated): Acid. sal. for rheumatic pains in 'small' joints; Apis mel. (acute dosage) for a sudden, hot swelling of the joint and a taut, shiny appearance; Bryonia for a dry, stiff 'cracking' joint that worsens with movement; Calc. carb. for a stiff, overweight, lethargic cat; Causticum for a stiff, old cat who may also be becoming senile; Caulophyllum for arthritis in knee, hock and other 'small' joints; and Rhus tox., the 'classic' remedy for typical symptoms that worsen in cold, damp weather and after rest.

herbal medicine

Feverfew, Devil's claw, Comfrey, Yucca, Cleavers, Burdock, Yarrow, Alfalfa, White-willow bark, and the 'greenleaf' herbs (Nettle, Parsley, Dandelion and Watercress) may be given as infusions. Many of these are also available in tablet form.

Bach flowers

Crabapple is an excellent cleansing remedy for toxins in the joints; Hornbeam will enhance strength.

acupuncture

Arthritis is particularly responsive to acupuncture treatment.

minor therapies

biochemical tissue salts

Ferr. phos. (acute dosage) is suitable for sudden-onset, acute arthritis;

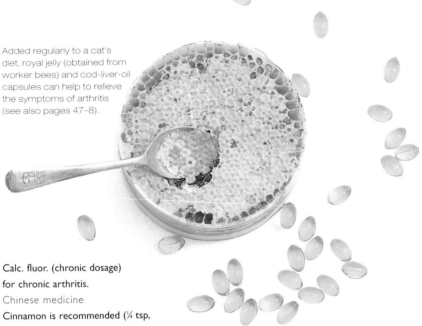

Added regularly to a cat's diet, royal jelly (obtained from worker bees) and cod-liver-oil capsules can help to relieve the symptoms of arthritis (see also pages 47–8).

Calc. fluor. (chronic dosage) for chronic arthritis.

Chinese medicine

Cinnamon is recommended (¼ tsp, powdered, to be given weekly).

crystals and gems

Ruby (liquid-gem remedy) may be given by mouth or added to water.

osteopathy and chiropractic

Some forms of arthritis – especially of the spine – generally benefit from and will respond well to both these forms of manipulation.

supplements

The following are all effective: kelp; cider vinegar, 5 ml (1 tsp) per 600 ml (1 pt) of drinking water; Vitamin C (250 mg daily); cod-liver oil (300 mg daily for one week, every four weeks); green-lipped-mussel extract (at half the recommended human dosage rate); B-complex vitamins (10 mg daily); and Vitamin E (50 iu daily). Royal jelly is extremely beneficial: 100 mg should be given daily. A copper collar can also be very beneficial for arthritis.

Causticum relieves arthritis

Dotty was an elderly, arthritic cat belonging to an equally mature and arthritic owner. Dotty was becoming progressively more stiff, and also more senile. She would somtimes stop and stare into space as though in a trance, and then 'come to', looking around as though surprised to find herself wherever she was.

I recommended the homoeopathic remedy Causticum, and mentioned to Dotty's owner that, in an old homoeopathic textbook of mine, this particular remedy was described as suiting 'broken-down old seniles'. Despite this rather impolite description, the causticum proved immensely beneficial for Dotty. She was visibly less stiff after taking the remedy twice a day for two weeks, and was subsequently given one dose twice weekly. Although still somewhat vacant at times, she is now much more mobile, and obviously feels fewer aches and pains.

sprains and strains

Pulled muscles, inflamed tendons, stretched ligaments: a whole range of minor injuries falls under the heading of sprains and strains. The usual human treatment of support bandaging and rest is often impossible to implement with a cat, who may also use a damaged joint or muscle too soon and aggravate the injury. However, natural medicines can often be extremely helpful.

Signs and symptoms Lameness, pain and sometimes an obvious swelling of the affected area.

aromatherapy
Rosemary, Juniper or Birch can be massaged into the region of the strain or sprain.

homoeopathy
Arnica (acute dosage) should be given as quickly as possible, followed by Ruta grav. (chronic dosage). Rhus tox. (chronic dosage) is beneficial for persistent lameness following a sprain or strain.

herbal medicine
Mallow, given as an infusion, will help to relieve the symptoms.

acupuncture
A course of acupuncture treatment is often rapidly effective, reducing the discomfort and any swelling, and assisting a rapid recovery.

minor therapies
biochemical tissue salts
Ferr. phos. alternated with Nat. phos. (acute dosage) is ideal for a recent sprain or strain; Mag. phos. alternating with Calc. phos. (chronic dosage) is suitable for a longer-term problem.

T-touch massage
A course of T-touch massage, as with acupuncture, will help to relieve pain and promote a quick recovery.

In T-touch massage, gentle circular movements are made randomly over the cat's body. These are said to generate specific brainwave patterns, instilling calmness and allowing natural healing to take place more rapidly (see also pages 30–1).

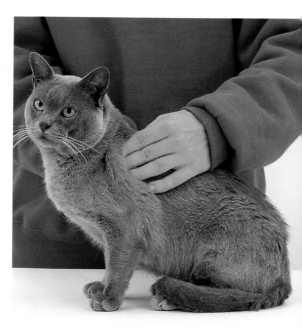

joint dislocation

In the cat, the hips are the most likely joints to become dislocated, and this often occurs through injury in road-traffic accidents. Physical replacement of a dislocated joint by a vet will be necessary, but natural remedies will help to prevent recurrence (a joint may easily redislocate due to the damage caused to the ligaments).

Signs and symptoms Obvious and sometimes dramatic lameness: an affected cat may even be unable to move. The dislocated joint may also be visibly misshapen.

homoeopathy
Rhus tox. and Ruta grav. should be given alternately (chronic dosage).

minor therapies
biochemical tissue salts
Calc. fluor. (acute dosage) may help.

supplements
Vitamin C is well-known for its role in accelerating the healing process of damaged tissue, and for promoting strong joints; it can also help to prevent recurrent dislocation. Add 250 mg to the diet daily.

bone fracture

Bone fractures may be 'closed' (with unbroken skin), or 'open' (the broken bone penetrates the skin). They are also classified as simple (one straightforward break) or comminuted (in several pieces). Fractures are usually caused by accidents, but can be spontaneous in thin or brittle bones. A fracture needs immediate treatment – sometimes with surgery – but natural medicines can play an important role in aiding recovery.

Signs and symptoms Obvious pain and lameness; a misshapen appearance; swelling around the fracture; you may hear the broken bones grating, or see them sticking out of the skin (an 'open' fracture).

homoeopathy
Arnica will minimize bruising and tissue damage; Symphytum hastens healing (both in acute dosage).

herbal medicine
Comfrey may be given as an infusion daily for two weeks to assist healing.

acupuncture
This often produces excellent results.

minor therapies
biochemical tissue salts
Calc. fluor. alternated with Calc. phos. (chronic dosage) will speed healing and strengthen bones.

supplements
As with joint dislocation (see above), adding Vitamin C to the diet of a cat who has suffered a bone fracture will promote rapid healing: 250 mg should be given daily.

myositis

  Myositis (muscle inflammation) is a painful condition that may be caused by infection, injury or disease of the immune system. While it can affect all muscles, a particularly severe form affects jaw muscles.
Signs and symptoms The affected muscle may become swollen and hard, and will be very tender to the touch.

homoeopathy

Aconite (acute dosage) is effective if it can be administered at an early stage. This treatment should be followed by Rhus tox. alternating with Bryonia (both given in chronic dosage). Causticum (chronic dosage) will alleviate any remaining stiffness.

herbal medicine

Feverfew is best given in the form of fresh leaves (one fresh leaf three times daily), although many cats may object to the bitter taste.

minor therapies

biochemical tissue salts

Ferr. phos. (acute dosage) will be helpful if it can be given at an early stage; this should be followed by Nat. phos. alternated with Mag. phos. (both in chronic dosage).

Chinese medicine

Black soybeans may be given in the form of infusions.

Feverfew has a natural anti-inflammatory action, reducing swelling and discomfort.

spondylosis

  This occurs when extra bone is laid down around the spinal vertebrae. The new bone may grow until it meets and fuses with an adjacent vertebra, and may press on the nerves leaving the spinal cord, resulting in pain and interference with nerve function. Spondylosis is mainly a condition of the older cat. The cause is usually unknown, but too much vitamin A in the diet may be a factor.
Signs and symptoms An inflexible and painful spine, with weakness or paralysis of one or more legs.

homoeopathy

Hypericum (chronic dosage) is effective for the pain resulting from pressure on the nerves; Causticum is useful for 'tearing' pains, and for stiffness in an older cat.

acupuncture

This treatment is often beneficial.

minor therapies

biochemical tissue salts

Calc. fluor. should be administered alternately with Calc. phos. (both in chronic dosage).

osteopathy and chiropractic

These manipulative treatments are both very beneficial in most cases of spondylosis.

osteomyelitis

This is an infection within bone. As antibiotics cannot penetrate bone easily, osteomyelitis can be serious and difficult to cure. It may occur following a bone fracture (see page 87).

Signs and symptoms Pain, fever and swelling; there may sometimes be a discharge of pus.

homoeopathy

Aconite (acute dosage) is effective if given early, especially if fever is also present. Hepar sulph. (acute dosage) is a good anti-infective remedy.

minor therapies
biochemical tissue salts

Calc. fluor. should be administered alternately with Calc. phos. (both in chronic dosage). If the infection within the bone persists, Calc. sulph. (also in chronic dosage) should be added to the first two tissue salts. As the infection begins to clear, Calc. carb. is suitable for the heavier cat, while Calc. phos. is suitable for the lighter cat and will help to strengthen the bone (both to be administered in chronic dosage).

osteoporosis

Thinning of the bones in a cat is unlikely to be due to a lack of oestrogen – as in humans – but to other metabolic malfunctions. However, the effects are similar. Osteoporosis may be caused by too much phosphorus and too little calcium and/or protein in the diet, by chronic kidney failure, and by lack of movement, resulting in weaker bones and joints.

Signs and symptoms An obvious unwillingness to move about, general weakness and an increased susceptibility to bone fractures (see page 87).

homoeopathy

The following are beneficial (all to be administered in chronic dosage): Calc. carb. for a well-built, obese cat; Calc. phos. for a slimmer and more active cat; and Silicea to strengthen the skeleton.

herbal medicine

Comfrey is also colloquially known as 'bone-knit', and – as this name suggests – is well-known in herbal folklore as a remedy for healing and strengthening bones. This herb should be given in the form of an infusion once weekly for a period of six weeks, in order to achieve the maximum benefit.

minor therapies
biochemical tissue salts

Calc. fluor. should be administered alternately with Calc. phos. (both in chronic dosage).

nervous system

This section covers diseases of the brain and nerves; behavioural problems commonly found in cats are dealt with separately (see pages 120–5).

The brain and nervous system are the command and control system for the body. From receiving information via sensory organs such as the eyes and ears, to organizing the control of muscle contractions and regulating heartbeats, the nervous system is integral to body function.

convulsions

Convulsions, or fits, are very frightening to witness. Epilepsy (one, but not the only, cause of convulsions) is the result of abnormal brain activity. Other causes include ingestion of certain poisons (such as anti-freeze – see also page 58), infection (such as tetanus – see page 119), metabolic disorders, injury or a brain tumour. A cat who is undergoing a fit should be kept as quiet as possible, ideally in a darkened room.

Signs and symptoms In a non-epileptic fit the cat will have muscle tremors, rigidity, loss of balance and muscle spasms. An epileptic fit is similar, but there may be confusion before and after the fit. Weakness, restlessness and a need to eat or drink are also typical.

aromatherapy
Lavender, Sweet marjoram and Camomile may be given by infusion, either after a fit or between fits.

homoeopathy
Cocculus (chronic dosage) is a general preventive remedy. Tarentula hisp. (chronic dosage) is helpful for a cat who is 'twitchy' after or between fits. The following may be given after a fit: Belladonna (acute dosage) if the pupils remain dilated; Cicuta virosa if the head was stretched back or to the side during the fit (acute dosage after the fit, then chronic dosage); Bufo (chronic dosage) if fits start during sleep; and Stramonium (acute dosage) if the cat falls to the left side.

herbal medicine
Skullcap with Valerian may be given either as an infusion or in tablet form. Hops, Rosemary, or Valerian with Melissa (Lemon balm) may also be given by infusion.

Bach flowers
Chestnut bud is a useful remedy.

minor therapies
biochemical tissue salts
Kali phos. (chronic dosage) may help.
Chinese medicine
Dates (½ tsp, chopped, daily) are recommended.
crystals and gems
Diamond (liquid-gem remedy) may be given by mouth or added to water.

neuritis

Inflammation of a nerve, or of a group of nerves, will lead to excessive discomfort in the area of tissue supplied by that nerve or nerves. For example, a persistent, localized itchiness may be due to inflammation of the nerve supplying that part of the skin.

Possible causes of neuritis are injuries (including surgical wounds), bacterial and viral infections, pressure (such as that caused by a 'trapped' or 'pinched' nerve), or the presence of a tumour.

Signs and symptoms Persistent localized pain or irritation, resulting in constant licking, scratching or biting at the affected area.

aromatherapy
Lavender may be massaged into the skin to relieve irritation.

homoeopathy
The following are helpful (all given in chronic dosage): Passiflora is a general soothing remedy; Chamomilla is suitable for an irritable cat; and Hypericum is ideal where there is physical damage at a nerve ending, such as at the site of a cut or bruise.

herbal medicine
Passiflora may be given by infusion.

Bach flowers
Star of Bethlehem may be beneficial.

minor therapies
biochemical tissue salts
Mag. phos. (chronic dosage) will help.
crystals and gems
Sapphire (liquid-gem remedy) may be given by mouth or added to water.

encephalitis and meningitis

These serious diseases both affect the brain. Encephalitis is an inflammation within the brain tissue; meningitis is an inflammation of the tissues around the brain. Causes include feline spongioform encephalopathy, bacterial or viral infections, or a tumour.

Signs and symptoms Pain, behavioural changes, hindleg paralysis, swaying, falling and fits.

aromatherapy
Lavender may be given by massage.

homoeopathy
Belladonna may be given if the pupils are dilated; Cuprum met. for muscle twitchings; and Stramonium if the cat falls to the left (all in acute dosage).

herbal medicine
Sage and Thyme are both useful when administered as infusions.

Bach flowers
Rock rose may help to alleviate the shock and fear associated with both conditions.

chorea

Chorea is an involuntary twitching of the muscles. It usually occurs in cats following a viral infection, but can also be caused by poisoning, or by a tumour in the brain.

Signs and symptoms Uncontrollable twitching, particularly of the limbs and facial muscles.

aromatherapy
Lavender may be used for massage.

homoeopathy
The following are helpful (all to be given in chronic dosage): Agaricus for post-viral chorea symptoms; Causticum for an old, stiff cat; and Conium if the hindquarters are weak.

herbal medicine
Skullcap with Valerian may be administered either as infusions or in tablet form. Rue, Rosemary, Oats and Lily-of-the-valley may all be used as infusions.

Bach flowers
Scleranthus may help to control the muscle twitchings.

minor therapies
biochemical tissue salts
Kali phos. (chronic dosage) may help.
Chinese medicine
One chicken-egg yolk should be added to the diet twice weekly.
crystals and gems
Diamond (liquid-gem remedy) may be given by mouth or added to water.

Agaricus improves chorea

Bertie was a cat who had suffered some form of minor brain damage (the cause was never ascertained, but may have been injury or a viral infection). Although he was fit and well, his head and body twitched uncontrollably as he walked.

This chorea had resisted all treatment, until I prescribed homoeopathic Agaricus. Given twice daily, this considerably alleviated the twitching within a week. The dosage was then reduced to alternate days, and subsequently to twice a week, with continued improvement. So far, Bertie continues to do well.

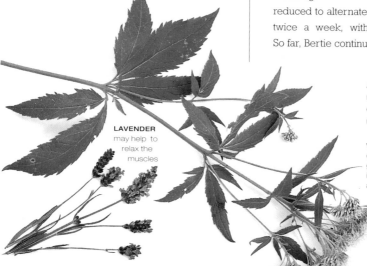

Although natural medicines may not be able to eliminate chorea entirely, they can be effective at reducing the muscle twitching.

LAVENDER may help to relax the muscles

VALERIAN is a natural calming agent. It is usually given with Skullcap to help in relieving restlessness and twitching

Key Gaskell syndrome

Key Gaskell syndrome is a mysterious condition named after the two people (Mr Key and Mr Gaskell) who first described the disease. It is also known as feline dysautonomia. The condition appeared several years ago and affected thousands of cats at the time. It now occurs only sporadically, but may well be a disease that could become epidemic again in the future.

Although it is a disease of the nervous system, only some nerves are affected. The nerves in question are the autonomic, or involuntary, nerves, over which the body has no conscious control – such as those that dictate whether the pupils are dilated or constricted, or those that control the bowel muscles whose function is to push food along.

Toxic chemicals in flea sprays or in food were considered a possible cause, but this has never been proved. Intensive nursing and support (particularly encouragement to eat) are essential for a cat suffering from Key Gaskell syndrome.

Signs and symptoms These include general dullness, dilated pupils, a dry mouth, loss of appetite, an inability to swallow food, constipation and vomiting (see page 97).

aromatherapy

Basil and Sweet marjoram will improve the weak and depressed state of a cat who is suffering from this condition.

homoeopathy

The following are beneficial (all to be given in chronic dosage): Gelsemium for the nerve and muscle weakness; Opium for the nerve weakness and constipation – Opium addicts suffer from constipation, so homoeopathic Opium will help to relieve it; and Belladonna for a dry mouth and dilated pupils.

Bach flowers

Olive is an ideal remedy for physical and mental exhaustion. Wild rose and Gorse are suitable for a cat who appears to be succumbing to the condition; and Clematis for a cat who goes into a 'dream world'.

minor therapies

biochemical tissue salts

Kali phos. is the biochemical nerve nutrient, and therefore suitable for use in a case of Key Gaskell syndrome; Nat. mur. is helpful when the affected cat has a dry mouth and constipation, and is in a weakened condition (both remedies to be given in chronic dosage).

Chinese medicine

Chinese food medicine recommends adding one cherry, chopped, to the cat's food daily.

crystals and gems

Liquid-remedy Ruby may be given by mouth or added to drinking water.

digestive system

This system starts – naturally enough – in the mouth, where it includes the teeth and any associated gum and dental disorders, as well as abnormalities of the salivary glands. The stomach and intestines, and all their possible problems, come next, followed by the liver and the pancreas, both of which are closely associated with digestion. The digestive system finishes at the rectum, and includes lower-bowel problems such as constipation and diarrhoea.

diseased teeth

 As a cat's diet is low in sugary foods, the likelihood of dental decay is small. However, the teeth do become diseased in other ways: for example, as a result of infection following damage, or due to gum erosion. Any conventional dental work carried out by your vet will be assisted by the natural remedies below.

Signs and symptoms Pain on eating, lack of appetite, drooling, loose or damaged teeth and halitosis.

homoeopathy for halitosis

Bruce was not nice to know. His halitosis (bad breath) was a feature that could not be ignored, and he became ostracized not only by the humans but even by the other cats with whom he was living.

Bruce became increasingly morose as his dental condition deteriorated, because his bad breath was caused by a combination of bad teeth and gum disease. His discomfort was also making him reluctant to eat.

A course of Hepar sulph. (given three times daily for one week) followed by Merc. sol. (twice daily for two weeks) greatly improved the situation. Although still not too pleasant at very close quarters, the aroma was diminished to a much more acceptable level.

Dental treatment carried out under a general anaesthetic to remove a few badly diseased teeth completed the process, and Bruce has now happily returned to the family fold.

homoeopathy

The following will be beneficial for a cat with damaged or diseased teeth (all to be administered in chronic dosage): Hepar sulph. will help to fight infection; Merc. sol. will control bad breath and excessive drooling of saliva; and Hypericum will relieve the pain that is caused by diseased teeth. This ability of Hypericum to relieve pain is an important one, as a cat who is experiencing even mild mouth pain may well refuse to eat. Liquidizing your cat's food, or adding a little water or gravy, will also make it softer and so easier to eat.

minor therapies

biochemical tissue salts

Calc. fluor. (chronic dosage) helps to strengthen teeth, and also increases resistance to infection and decay.

gingivitis and stomatitis

Gingivitis (or gum inflammation) and stomatitis (inflammation of the mouth lining) often occur together, or one may lead to the other. These conditions may be associated with diseased teeth, or they may result from infection, poisoning or kidney disease (see page 104). Any necessary conventional dental treatment should be followed by a raw-food-based diet to help to prevent recurrence.

Signs and symptoms Reddened gums, mouth ulcers, obvious pain on eating, bad breath and excessive drooling.

aromatherapy
Terebinth and Lavender essential oils may be used for massage.

homoeopathy
The following will give symptomatic relief (acute dosage in early stages; chronic dosage for a longstanding case): Acid. nit. or Borax for gingivitis with mouth ulcers; Belladonna for a very reddened mouth and a feverish patient; Merc. cor. for pain and profuse salivation; and Phosphorus for bleeding gums.

herbal medicine
Echinacea, Myrrh or Goldenseal, in the form of a tincture, may be applied directly to the gums and mouth. Sage and Rosemary may be given by infusion. Garlic is a good remedy, and should be given as ⅓ chopped clove daily, or alternated with 250 mg Vitamin C.

minor therapies
biochemical tissue salts
Calc. sulph. (acute dosage) is ideal for swollen and bleeding gums.
Chinese medicine
Persimmon (sharon fruit) and star fruit may be beneficial: ⅓ of each, chopped, should be given daily.
crystals and gems
Emerald (liquid-gem remedy) may be given by mouth or added to water.

salivary cyst

A swelling in the facial area is often assumed to be an abscess, but a saliva-filled cyst is another possibility. The cause of such cysts is unknown. Surgical drainage is normally required, and may need to be repeated if the cyst subsequently refills.

Signs and symptoms The appearance of a soft facial swelling that increases in size.

homoeopathy
Apis mel. is helpful for a soft swelling that 'pits' on pressure; Phytolacca is suitable for a firm swelling; and Silicea may be used at a later stage if the swelling hardens (all in acute dosage).

pharyngitis

Pharyngitis is, essentially, a sore throat – and everyone knows how painful that can be. The condition in cats may occur due to viral, bacterial or fungal infections, after swallowing certain irritant poisons, or because a foreign body of some kind has become lodged in the pharynx (the throat).

Signs and symptoms Persistent coughing, retching, lack of appetite and enlarged lymph glands beneath the jaw.

aromatherapy
Bergamot, Hyssop, Sage and Thyme will all provide relief when gently massaged into the throat area.

homoeopathy
Baryta carb. is ideal for a young cat with pharyngitis and swollen lymph glands; Lachesis for a very inflamed, purplish throat; and Phytolacca for a painful throat with enlarged lymph glands (all in chronic dosage).

herbal medicine
Echinacea tincture will be soothing if given by mouth three times daily.

Bach flowers
Star of Bethlehem is a good remedy for a 'tense' throat.

minor therapies
biochemical tissue salts
Calc. phos. is suitable for pharyngitis with tonsillitis; Calc. sulph. will

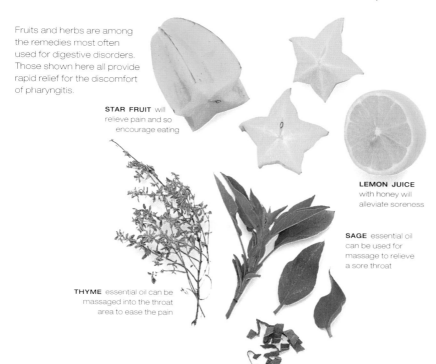

Fruits and herbs are among the remedies most often used for digestive disorders. Those shown here all provide rapid relief for the discomfort of pharyngitis.

STAR FRUIT will relieve pain and so encourage eating

LEMON JUICE with honey will alleviate soreness

SAGE essential oil can be used for massage to relieve a sore throat

THYME essential oil can be massaged into the throat area to ease the pain

soothe a painful, ulcerated throat; and Ferr. phos. is helpful for pharyngitis that is accompanied by laryngitis (all in chronic dosage).
Chinese medicine
Lemon juice should be given at the rate of 2.5 ml (½ tsp) with a little

honey twice daily. Star fruit will also help to alleviate the soreness and encourage eating: ⅓ of the chopped fruit should be added to food daily.
crystals and gems
Sapphire (liquid-gem remedy) may be given by mouth or added to water.

vomiting

Occasional vomiting in cats is not unusual, and can be treated effectively with natural medicines. Common causes include viral and bacterial infections, eating inappropriate foods, poisoning, a foreign body, stomach or intestinal abnormalities, liver and pancreatic disease (see page 99) and kidney disease (see page 104).

Do not feed a cat for 24 hours after vomiting has occurred, and then feed a bland diet for at least two days (see page 101).

Signs and symptoms Unmissable! If a cat is vomiting frequently or continuously, vomiting blood, or vomiting with other acute symptoms, he or she must be examined by a vet as soon as possible.

aromatherapy
Mint, Lavender and Tarragon may all be given, by massage or diffuser.

homoeopathy
The following may be helpful (given in acute dosage for severe vomiting; and in chronic dosage for persistent vomiting): Arsen. alb. for vomiting with diarrhoea; Apomorphine for repeated vomiting, often as soon as food is swallowed; Ipecac. for intermittent vomiting with much retching; and Nux vomica for post-operative vomiting and after eating unsuitable foods.

herbal medicine
Infusions of Gentian root, St John's wort or Peppermint may be given.

minor therapies
biochemical tissue salts
The following are all effective remedies (to be given in acute dosage for severe vomiting, or in chronic dosage for a longstanding problem): Ferr. phos. for vomiting of undigested food; Kali mur. for vomiting of thick mucus, especially after eating fatty food; Nat. phos. when sour, acid vomit is produced and the patient is irritable; and Nat. sulph. for vomited bile.
Chinese medicine
Fennel seeds (½ tsp daily) and grated cloves (⅛ tsp daily) may be added to the cat's food.
crystals and gems
Emerald (liquid-gem remedy) may be given by mouth or added to water.

fur balls

 Some of the dead hair removed by self-grooming is inevitably swallowed. This may form a ball, which will irritate the stomach and cause the cat to vomit up the fur. In very rare cases, surgery may be required: I once removed a fur ball the size of an orange from a cat's stomach. Giving oily foods such as sardines is a good preventive measure, as is regular grooming (see also page 40).

Signs and symptoms Persistent vomiting or retching to no effect, and a reluctance to eat.

homoeopathy	minor therapies
Nux vomica (chronic dosage) or Ornithogallum tincture (acute dosage) will help to alleviate symptoms.	crystals and gems Emerald (liquid-gem remedy) may be given by mouth or added to water.

foreign bodies

 Unusual objects swallowed by a cat may become lodged in the oesophagus, stomach or – more commonly – in the intestines. If the foreign body is obstructing the intestine, surgery will be necessary; in other cases, the object may eventually pass through, or may be vomited up.

Signs and symptoms Vomiting, little or no passage of faeces, abdominal pain and lethargy.

homoeopathy	minor therapies
Colchicum or Nux vomica is suitable for a foreign body in the intestines; Ornithogallum tincture for a foreign body in the stomach (acute dosage).	crystals and gems Emerald can be effective: the liquid remedy may be given by mouth or added to drinking water.

intussusception

In this condition the intestine telescopes into itself due to excessive muscular movements of the bowel wall, resulting in a potentially serious obstruction. Surgery is normally required, but in the early stages natural remedies can be successful.

Signs and symptoms Vomiting, diarrhoea, straining and obvious abdominal pain.

homoeopathy	minor therapies
Colchicum and Nux vomica should be given alternately (acute dosage).	crystals and gems Liquid-remedy Emerald may be given.

liver disease

 The liver has a variety of functions, which include producing enzymes needed for digestion (in bile), controlling the distribution of nutrients around the body, and detoxifying poisons. Liver disease may be acute (as in hepatitis) or chronic (as in cirrhosis). Causes include bacterial and viral infections, poisoning, tumours and obstruction of the bile duct.

Signs and symptoms Vomiting, weight loss, lethargy, ascites (see page 76) and jaundice.

aromatherapy

Mint with Rosemary is ideal for acute liver disease; Wild marjoram with Rosemary for chronic liver disease.

herbal medicine

Blue flag, Centaury, Southernwood, Dandelion or Yellow dock may be given as infusions.

homoeopathy

The following are effective (all given in chronic dosage): Carduus for cirrhosis, a swollen liver and ascites (see page 76); Chelidonium for jaundice; Lycopodium for digestive problems and flatulence; Nux vomica for digestive upsets; and Phosphorus for pain and vomiting.

minor therapies

biochemical tissue salts

Nat. sulph. (chronic dosage) may help to alleviate the symptoms.

Chinese medicine

One plum should be diced and given on alternate days. In addition, ½ tsp each of chopped chicory and kohl rabi should be given daily.

pancreatitis

 There are two main types of pancreatic disease in cats: diabetes mellitus (see pages 82–3) and pancreatitis (inflammation of the pancreas), which is a very painful acute condition and a very debilitating chronic one. The causes are unknown, but may follow the use of steroids. Emergency treatment may be necessary in an acute case; otherwise the following remedies will help.

Signs and symptoms Obvious pain, fever, vomiting, diarrhoea and a lack of appetite.

homoeopathy

Phosphorus and Iris vers. (acute dosage) are both suitable remedies.

herbal medicine

Yarrow may be given as infusions.

minor therapies

biochemical tissue salts

Nat. phos. should be alternated with Ferr. phos. (acute dosage).

crystals and gems

Liquid-remedy Topaz may be given.

constipation

Cats suffer much less frequently from constipation than humans do. However, it is an occasional problem, and is no less uncomfortable for the feline species than it is for us. Constipation may be caused by a diet that is too low in fibre (roughage), by an enlarged or constricted lower bowel, or by the presence of polyps or tumours in the bowel.

Feeding a healthy, nutritionally balanced diet containing plenty of roughage – such as that obtained from raw vegetables, fruit, pulses, nuts and grains – will go a long way towards resolving constipation (see also page 44); the following remedies will also help.

Signs and symptoms Straining to defecate, producing thin, flattened faeces (or none at all), and long periods between bowel movements.

homoeopathy

The following should all be given in chronic dosage: Calc. carb. for large, bulky stools passed infrequently; Nux vomica for post-operative constipation, or after over-eating; Sepia for constipation associated with liver problems; and Silicea where the stool is almost passed, but then recedes into the rectum (often known as the 'shy-stool' syndrome).

herbal medicine

Rhubarb may be used as an infusion, or a small amount may be added to food. A decoction of Frangula bark is a gentle and efficacious remedy.

Bach flowers

Crabapple is well-known as the cleansing remedy, and often helps to relieve constipation.

minor therapies
biochemical tissue salts

The following may also be used (all in chronic dosage): Calc. fluor. for a completely inactive bowel; Kali mur. for constipation following over-eating or eating very rich food; and Nat. mur. for constipation alternating with diarrhoea. Nat. phos. and Nat. sulph. may also be given alternately for persistent constipation.

Chinese medicine

White radish is helpful: this should be finely chopped, and ½ tsp mixed with food daily.

crystals and gems

Ruby (liquid-gem remedy) may be given by mouth or added to water.

supplements

Bran, dried fruit and psyllium husks are very effective ingredients of a high-fibre diet. Liquid paraffin (5 ml [1 tsp] daily by mouth) will lubricate and loosen for short periods, and often provides rapid relief from constipation. However, paraffin does prevent the Vitamins A, D, E and K from being absorbed by the body, and persistent use will result in vitamin deficiency, so always consult your vet before giving it to your cat.

diarrhoea

Diarrhoea can vary from mild symptoms, where a cat simply has loose faeces, to acute colitis (inflammation of the colon), where the patient is extremely unwell and passes blood and mucus. The causes are many, including sudden dietary change, stress, liver malfunction, parasites and tumours.

Withholding food for 24 hours may solve the problem; bland foods (such as chicken, fish and pasta) should then be given for at least two days, before gradually returning to the usual diet.

Signs and symptoms Abnormal stool consistency (ranging from semi-solid to watery), possibly with blood, mucus or undigested food. The cat may strain a great deal, and may need to defecate very frequently.

aromatherapy
Cinnamon may be used for massage.

homoeopathy
The following will be helpful (acute dosage for sudden diarrhoea; chronic dosage for long-term diarrhoea): Aloe vera for flatulence and mucus; Arsen. alb. for food poisoning (with vomiting); Chamomilla for frothy diarrhoea; Colocynth for diarrhoea with pain and an arched back; Merc. sol. for loose stools; Nux vomica after eating bad food; phosphorus for straining, with mucus and/or blood; and Podophyllum for watery faeces.

herbal medicine
Arrowroot, Catechu, dried Bilberries, Meadowsweet, Plantain and Slippery elm may be given. Slippery elm is available in tablet form; the other herbs may be given as infusions.

Bach flowers
For stress-related diarrhoea, Impatiens is helpful for an irritable cat; Aspen for an anxious one.

minor therapies
biochemical tissue salts
The following are all beneficial (acute dosage for acute or recent diarrhoea; chronic dosage for longstanding diarrhoea): Calc. phos. for pancreatic problems and malabsorption; Calc. sulph for frequent, gushing diarrhoea; Ferr. phos. for sudden diarrhoea in a young cat; Kali mur. for pale, loose stools; Kali phos. for diarrhoea in a stressed cat; Nat. mur. for diarrhoea alternating with constipation; Nat. phos. for sour, green diarrhoea; and Nat. sulph. for dark, runny stools.

Chinese medicine
Ginger (ground) or crabapple (chopped) should be given (½ tsp daily for one week). Ginseng may be given as tablets (25 mg daily), or as ¼ tsp of the diced root on alternate days for 10 days.

supplements
Live yoghurt should be given after an infection: this will help to repopulate the bowel with bacteria needed for normal bowel function. Add 5 ml (1 tsp) to each meal for one week.

urinary system

The bladder and kidneys, and their connections – the ureters and urethra – form the urinary system. Symptoms of bladder problems are usually very obvious, but signs of kidney disease may be more difficult to differentiate from those of other conditions, such as hyperthyroidism (see page 81) or diabetes mellitus (see pages 82–3) .

Urinary problems, such as cystitis and kidney failure, are all too common in cats. This may be partly because most cats drink very little, and so are predisposed to such conditions. One theory for this is that domestic cats are descended from desert cats, who had to learn to conserve fluid, and were rarely able to drink. Healthy kidneys are crucial – they remove waste products from the body and help to maintain water levels.

cystitis
This condition – in all animals – is far more common in the female than in the male, and cats are no exception. The causes are bacterial infection, the development of bladder 'stones' (see pages 104–5), injury or the presence of tumours.

Signs and symptoms Straining to pass urine frequently, with obvious discomfort, and blood appearing in the urine.

aromatherapy
Juniper, Sandalwood and Ylang ylang are all beneficial remedies for recurrent cystitis, and may be used for gentle massage.

homoeopathy
Cantharis (acute dosage) is suitable for acute, painful cystitis; Causticum, Equisetum and Thlaspi bursa (chronic dosage) for persistent cystitis.

herbal medicine
Buchu, Couchgrass, Dandelion, Uva ursi (often known as Bearberry), Parsley, Watercress and Horsetail may all be used as infusions.

Bach flowers
Rescue Remedy will help to relieve the discomfort of acute cystitis.

minor therapies
biochemical tissue salts
Ferr. phos. (administered in acute dosage) should be followed by Mag. phos. (administered in chronic dosage).

Chinese medicine
Hops are the recommended remedy for cystitis according to Chinese medicine: 1 tsp of these should be diced finely and added to the cat's food daily.

crystals and gems
Pearl (liquid-gem remedy) may be helpful in some cases. This may either be given by mouth or added to drinking water.

supplements
Vitamin C (administered at a rate of 250 mg daily), will promote a rapid recovery from cystitis.

feline urolithiasis syndrome In this condition,

tiny mineral crystals form in the urine, causing irritation that can trigger cystitis. The crystals may collect in the urethra (which carries urine away from the bladder), causing obstruction. If this prevents the passage of urine, the cat will need urgent veterinary attention.

Signs and symptoms This condition produces the same symptoms as a bout of cystitis (see opposite): obvious abdominal discomfort, and unsuccessful straining to pass urine.

aromatherapy

Juniper and Sandalwood essential oils may be used for massage.

homoeopathy

Thlaspi bursa will help to dissolve crystals in 'classic' FUS. Also useful are the following (all in chronic dosage): Benzoic acid, where the urine is dark and sweet-smelling; Calc. carb. for an obese, inactive cat; and Lycopodium if reddish-coloured, sandy material is passed out with the urine.

herbal medicine

Barberry root, Sarsaparilla root and Gravel root, given by decoction, may all help to relieve the symptoms.

Bach flowers

Crabapple is beneficial, especially if there is leakage of urine.

minor therapies

biochemical tissue salts

Nat. sulph. (chronic dosage) should be given.

Chinese medicine

Star fruit is advised: ⅓ fruit, chopped, should be added to food daily.

homoeopathy and a natural diet

George was a large cat. He weighed in at a hefty 9.1 kg (20 lb), which – even in spite of his sizable physique – would be classified as obese in feline terms. Just one of the many problems to which overweight cats are predisposed is feline urolithiasis syndrome, and this uncomfortable condition began to afflict George with a vengeance. Passing urine became a distressing procedure, and twice he become completely obstructed and had to be catheterized (this involves passing a fine tube up the urethra, which carries urine away from the bladder) in order to clear the blockage.

The natural-medicine approach that we adopted consisted of a two-pronged attack: a strict diet, and the homoeopathic remedy Thlaspi bursa. The diet – reluctantly adhered to by George's owner, and even more reluctantly by George himself – gradually reduced his weight to a trimmer 6.4 kg (14 lb). The Thlaspi bursa – a remedy obtained from a useful plant known as the Shepherd's purse – also seemed to help. This was given three times daily for one week, twice daily for two weeks, and then twice weekly for a further four weeks. The symptoms rapidly began to disappear, until George was once again able to pass urine freely and without discomfort.

kidney disease
There are many forms of kidney disease, ranging from acute, life-threatening kidney infections to 'wearing out' of the kidneys in old age. In addition to ageing, causes include bacterial or viral infections, poisoning and tumours. It is important to treat kidney disease in its early stages.

Signs and symptoms Increased thirst, weight loss and lack of appetite. Where the kidney disease is advanced, symptoms may also include weakness, vomiting, dehydration and oedema (see pages 76–7).

aromatherapy
Juniper may be used for massage.

homoeopathy
Phosphorus (acute dosage) will be beneficial for a cat suffering from acute kidney disease. Merc. sol. is suitable for a chronic condition with mouth ulcers, a wet mouth and increased thirst; Nat. mur. for increased thirst and poor skin condition (both in chronic dosage).

herbal medicine
Alfalfa, Cornsilk, Cleavers, Parsley and Parsnip may be given by infusion.

Bach flowers
Olive will help to alleviate weakness.

minor therapies
biochemical tissue salts
Ferr. phos. is suitable for acute kidney infection; Kali phos. for chronic kidney infection (both in acute dosage).
Chinese medicine
I tsp of ginger or watermelon peel, chopped, should be given daily.
crystals and gems
Diamond (liquid-gem remedy) may help: this may be given by mouth or added to drinking water.

urolithiasis
'Stones' may form in the bladder, or are occasionally found in the kidneys or urethra. They are composed of minerals in solution in the urine, which form crystals that coagulate to produce the 'stones'. Some are smooth, others are sharp and can cause intense discomfort. Urolithiasis may result from an imbalance in body fluids due to urine alkalinity or to an insufficient intake of water.

Signs and symptoms Blood in the urine, obvious abdominal pain (do not squeeze your cat's tummy) and incontinence.

aromatherapy
Juniper, Sandalwood and Ylang ylang are all suitable remedies, and may be used for gentle massage.

homoeopathy
The following may be beneficial (all in chronic dosage): Calc. carb. for an overweight cat; Calc. phos. for a

lighter, more active cat; Thlaspi bursa for a persistent tendency to produce small 'stones'; and Benzoic acid when the urine is dark and sweet-smelling.

herbal medicine

Birch leaves, Bearberry root and Couchgrass may be given as infusions, and Sarsaparilla root as decoctions. These will soothe an inflamed bladder and help to prevent stone formation.

minor therapies
biochemical tissue salts

Mag. phos. may alternated with Calc. phos.; alternatively, Nat. sulph. may be given (both in chronic dosage).

Chinese medicine

Star fruit (½ fresh fruit, chopped), should be added to food daily.

crystals and gems

Pearl (liquid-gem remedy) may be given by mouth or added to water.

incontinence

A cat who leaves wet patches during his or her sleep, or who dribbles urine at other times, is not an ideal companion. Bladder control is also extremely important for a cat's comfort and health. This condition has a number of causes, including cystitis (see page 102), bladder 'stones' (see opposite, below), tumours and spinal injury. Do not restrict your cat's water intake.

Signs and symptoms The urine leakage may be occasional, frequent, or almost continuous in a severely affected cat.

homoeopathy

Agnus castus is beneficial for an old male cat, and Baryta carb. for a very young or older cat of either sex. Causticum will help to strengthen weak bladder muscles, thereby reducing the leakage of urine. (All to be given in chronic dosage.)

minor therapies
biochemical tissue salts

Calc. phos. (chronic dosage) is ideal for incontinence in an old cat.

Chinese medicine

Chestnuts or liquorice (chopped), or cinnamon (powdered), may help: ½ tsp should be given daily to encourage normal bladder function.

reducing urine leakage

Ernest was a proud old Siamese. He was 17, but still the top cat among the four in the household, owning the rights to the warmest, most comfortable spot in the house – the airing cupboard. He still went out each morning, but, unfortunately, had succumbed to one problem of old age – incontinence. His slumbers in the cupboard invariably resulted in damp patches on the blankets. Things went from bad to worse, and Ernest seemed to leak constantly!

Happily, homoeopathy came to the rescue. Causticum and Agnus castus, given twice daily for three weeks, followed by Causticum only twice weekly, successfully reduced the urine leakage to a very occasional drip.

female reproductive system

It seems to be the lot of the female of the species to suffer from more problems and diseases of the reproductive system than the male. Many, but not all, of these are associated with pregnancy and the process of giving birth.

The reproductive system includes the ovaries, the uterus, and the mammary (milk) glands. Naturally, cats who are spayed (neutered) early in life will avoid most of the diseases of the reproductive system, although mammary problems can still occur, as can a condition called stump pyometra, in which the stump of the uterus left after spaying can become infected.

Unspayed cats, and in particular those used for breeding, are the individuals most likely to develop one of a whole range of reproductive system ailments.

metritis and pyometra

 Metritis is an inflammation of the uterus (womb); it is caused by infection, and usually occurs after pregnancy and birth. Pyometra is a form of metritis in which uterine secretions build up and become infected, due to a hormonal imbalance. If acute, both conditions are potentially life-threatening, and may necessitate an emergency hysterectomy.

 Signs and symptoms An unpleasant, smelly vaginal discharge (in a 'closed' pyometra, this may not occur), a high fever, increased thirst and loss of appetite.

aromatherapy
Sage may be used for massage.

homoeopathy
The following are beneficial (all in acute dosage unless specified): Caulophyllum for chocolate-coloured vaginal discharge; Helonias for hindquarter weakness; Hydrastis in early pyometra with a large amount of catarrhal discharge; Sabina when copious fresh blood is present in the discharge; and Sepia (chronic dosage) for persistent chronic metritis or pyometra.

herbal medicine
Goldenseal, Myrrh and Rose hips may all be given by infusion.

minor therapies
biochemical tissue salts
Ferr. phos. (acute dosage) should be given, followed by Calc. sulph. (chronic dosage).
Chinese medicine
The following are all recommended: ½ tsp of chive seed; 25 g (1 oz) yam; or 25 g (1 oz) mussels daily.
crystals and gems
Liquid-remedy Diamond may help.

mastitis

 Inflamed mammary glands are extremely uncomfortable for a cat. They can also be accompanied by a high fever, bringing a risk of major damage to the glands. The cause is usually bacterial infection (especially after pregnancy), or a mammary tumour.

Signs and symptoms Hot, swollen, painful glands; abscesses may also form, and the nipples may appear to be redder than normal.

homoeopathy

The following are all recommended (acute dosage): Belladonna for hot, painful glands and fever; Bryonia for hot, hard glands when the cat is unwilling to move; and Phytolacca (chronic dosage) for 'knotty' glands.

minor therapies
biochemical tissue salts
Ferr. phos. (acute dosage) will alleviate the symptoms at an early stage of mastitis. Silica (chronic dosage) should be given at a later stage, if the glands have become thickened and hardened.

Chinese medicine
A mixture of malt and crushed onion will be soothing if applied directly to the glands. Chopped radish leaf or malt (½ tsp daily) may also be added to food.

crystals and gems
Liquid-remedy Topaz may be given.

infertility

 In many instances, no specific cause can be found for a lack of fertility; it may simply result from an unsuccessful mating. Alternatively, it could be due to a combination of factors such as stress, obesity, hormonal imbalance, infections or abnormalities of the reproductive organs. The problem could, of course, also be with the tom cat.

Signs and symptoms A cat with fertility problems will either not become pregnant, or will produce only small litters.

homoeopathy
Sepia should be given alternately with Pulsatilla (chronic dosage). Platina (chronic dosage) may also be helpful.

herbal medicine
Raspberry-leaf, given by infusion or in tablet form, may help.

Bach flowers
Clematis should be given when a cat lacks energy; Larch is useful when a cat lacks self-confidence and is shy.

minor therapies
biochemical tissue salts
Nat. mur. (chronic dosage) is an effective remedy.

Chinese medicine
5 mg Ginseng may be given daily.

supplements
Royal jelly is a useful supplement.

abortion

This is the expulsion of foetuses from the mother's body before they are due to be born. Some cats suffer from repeated abortions; a pregnant cat may also re-absorb one or more foetuses, even some weeks into pregnancy.

Abortion may be due to infection, injury, hormonal imbalance or a nutritionally inadequate diet.

Signs and symptoms Vaginal discharge, ejection of the dead foetuses, lethargy, and dullness and depression.

homoeopathy

Viburnum opulis should be given in the first three weeks of pregancy, followed by Caulophyllum in the last six weeks of pregnancy (both in chronic dosage).

Bach flowers

Wild rose may help in a cat who has experienced previous abortions.

minor therapies

biochemical tissue salts

Calc. phos. is recommended (to be given in chronic dosage throughout the pregnancy).

Chinese medicine

To prevent abortion, Chinese medicine recommends feeding one chicken-egg yolk to the cat twice weekly, throughout the pregnancy.

dystocia

In general, cats have less difficulty in giving birth than we do, mainly because they usually have several small babies rather than one large one. Where problems do arise, the cause may be a hormonal imbalance, stress, or abnormalities in the foetuses. Natural medicines are extremely useful in promoting an easy labour and birth.

Signs and symptoms Straining for a long period, without producing kittens.

aromatherapy

Use Lavender and Sage for gentle massage several days before birth and during labour if problems arise.

homoeopathy

Caulophyllum is beneficial during pregnancy (chronic dosage) and the birth (acute dosage). After the birth, Arnica (acute dosage) will reduce bruising around the vulva.

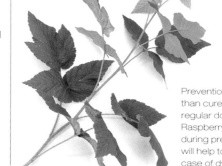

Prevention is better than cure, and a regular dose of Raspberry leaf during pregnancy will help to avert a case of dystocia.

herbal medicine

Raspberry leaf should be given by infusion or tablets during pregnancy, to assist a straightforward labour.

Bach flowers

Walnut may be given throughout pregnancy. At the time of labour, oak will encourage a cat who has stopped straining to 'try harder'; Star of Bethlehem will encourage straining if the cat has stopped in fear or panic.

minor therapies
biochemical tissue salts

Administer Calc. fluor. alternately with Kali phos. during a difficult labour (both in acute dosage).

Bach remedies calm mother

Annabel was a rather disdainful Siamese. Pregnancy did not suit her – she obviously resented the extra weight. As for the messy business of giving birth – too much to bear. One kitten appeared after desultory straining, and the effect was instant: the owner described an expression of utter panic on Annabel's face. She ignored the kitten, stopped straining, and began a Siamese nervous breakdown.

I recommended the Bach remedies Star of Bethlehem (for panic), Oak (for greater effort) and Willow (for resentment: in this case, of the kitten), with one drop of each to be given every five minutes for 30 minutes. By then Annabel had calmed down, began straining again and eventually produced four healthy kittens.

agalactia

This condition arises when a new mother has inadequate milk for her kittens. Either too little milk or no milk at all may be produced as a result of a hormonal imbalance, stress or mastitis (see page 107).
Signs and symptoms A litter of hungry, noisy kittens usually reveals agalactia very rapidly!

Fennel is one of several herbs that have a natural ability to stimulate milk production.

homoeopathy
Calc. phos. or Lecithin (acute dosage).

herbal medicine
Milk wort, Goat's rue and Fennel all have a milk-producing capacity.

Bach flowers
Crabapple is a good remedy.

minor therapies
biochemical tissue salts

Kali mur. (acute dosage) may help.

Chinese medicine
Small amounts (I tsp daily) of the following foods, given for a few days, will help to encourage the formation of milk: dill seed, asparagus, lettuce seed, and chicken with ginger and dried shrimp.

crystals and gems
Liquid-remedy Ruby may be given.

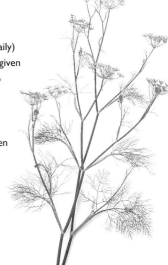

male reproductive system

The male of the species is luckier than the female in that diseases of his reproductive system are few and far between. Male cats are also luckier than their human and canine counterparts in that they have no prostate gland, which can be a source of great discomfort and distress to many older men and dogs.

Only two conditions in male cats are seen by vets on a regular basis, one of which, orchitis, causes great anxiety to an affected cat. The other, hypersexuality, causes more distress to those around him! Hypersexuality is, in essence, a natural hormone drive that is out of control, or is so pronounced as to have anti-social effects.

hypersexuality

The only cure for uncontrollable hypersexuality in a male cat may be castration, but natural medicines can often be beneficial. Hypersexual behaviour may be the result of a hormonal imbalance, or of habitual learned behaviour (just as children learn and continue bad habits, so cats can begin acting anti-socially, and then find that they cannot stop).

Signs and symptoms Aggression displayed towards other cats (especially over territorial rights), roaming and urine-spraying; the testicles may also be swollen.

aromatherapy
Lavender and Sweet marjoram, used for massage, will both have a calming, soothing influence.

homoeopathy
The following are good remedies (all to be administered in chronic dosage): Cantharis, especially if the hypersexuality is accompanied by an irritable bladder; Phosphorus for a cat who is particularly nervous and excitable; Tarentula hisp. for a hysterical cat who is liable to bite; and Ustillago maydis for a cat who has swollen testicles and is very active sexually.

herbal medicine
Skullcap with Valerian, or Hops, may be given by infusion. Both of these remedies should produce a calming effect, and therefore lessen the risk of aggressive behaviour.

Bach flowers
Vervain is suitable for an 'over-enthusiastic' male cat; Impatiens will often help to relax an irritable and excitable individual.

minor therapies
biochemical tissue salts
Mag. phos. (given in chronic dosage) may be helpful.

orchitis

 Orchitis is inflammation of the testicles, and is one of the most painful conditions to affect male cats. This disorder may be caused by injury, a bacterial infection or a tumour.

Signs and symptoms Obviously painful, swollen testicles, frequent licking of the testicles, and possible difficulty in passing urine. The pain may become so acute that the cat will stop eating, will be reluctant to move and may cry out with pain. If the inflammation spreads, he may find it difficult to pass any urine at all. If infection is present, the cat may become feverish and weak, and there will be a danger of septicaemia (blood poisoning): seek veterinary help urgently.

orchitis cured with homoeopathy

The biggest, strongest, most bullying tom for miles around, Sam was in no danger of being challenged for the position of top cat. He was the only entire (unneutered) male cat living in the area, and appeared to relish reminding everyone of the fact.

Sam had the strongest smell that I have known in a tom cat, and spread this around liberally. His owner either had no sense of smell, or no sense of civic duty, since Sam would urine-mark his vast territory at every possible opportunity, to the discontent of the whole neighbourhood.

However, after suffering an injury of some kind, Sam was brought to my surgery with bruised, blackened and swollen testicles that were obviously causing him considerable pain. Homoeopathy came to the rescue: I prescribed Belladonna to reduce the inflammation, and Arnica for the bruising and trauma (both to be administered in acute dosage). This treatment rapidly brought the condition of Sam's testicles back to normal, and within three days he was pursuing his usual habits. Sam's owner thanked me profusely, although – strangely enough – no-one else did.

homoeopathy

Belladonna (acute dosage) is often beneficial where intense pain and heat are present, and when the testicles are sensitive to the slightest touch; Bryonia (acute dosage) is a good remedy where the testicles have become hardened and there is pain (gently pressing on the testicles will also provide relief). Where the testicles are hardened and perhaps scarred, Rhododendron (chronic dosage) should be given.

minor therapies

biochemical tissue salts

Ferr. phos. (acute dosage) will help to relieve the swelling.

Chinese medicine

Kelp powder is the recommended remedy in Chinese medicine for a case of orchitis: the powder should be added to the diet at a dosage rate of 1 tsp daily.

crystals and gems

Sapphire (liquid-gem remedy) is often beneficial: this may either be given by mouth or added to the affected cat's drinking water.

cancer

Cancerous tissue, or tumours, can grow in any tissue or part of any body organ. Some tumours – such as skin tumours – are obvious, but others may go unnoticed until they are quite advanced. Cancer seems to be increasing in incidence in cats, perhaps because they are now living longer. It is also surprisingly common in young cats, especially when linked with infections such as the feline leukaemia and feline immunodeficiency viruses (see page 118). Natural remedies can contain and sometimes cure cancer, and will help to relieve the symptoms even in a terminal case.

aromatherapy

Rosemary and Ylang ylang will be revitalizing when used to massage an old cat afflicted with cancer.

homoeopathy

Hydrastis will help in an early case of cancer, while Arsen. alb. relieves pain and suffering in terminal cancer (both in acute dosage). Echinacea (chronic dosage) assists the immune system in fighting cancer. Viscum alb. (chronic dosage), the homoeopathic remedy made from mistletoe, is also beneficial in most cases.

herbal medicine

Good results have been obtained by giving Mistletoe extract by injection. Echinacea tincture, and infusions of Red clover and Autumn crocus may also be used. Apricot kernels, ground and refrigerated, and given at a dose rate of 25 mg daily, have been shown to be beneficial (the kernels must not be kept in water, as this can cause a reaction that will liberate a toxin).

Bach flowers

Crabapple is an excellent general cleansing remedy. Other effective treatments include the following: Hornbeam, to give strength to a weakened cat; Mimulus for a cat who seems to be frightened by his or her symptoms; and Olive, to aid a cat who appears to have lost the will to live.

minor therapies

biochemical tissue salts

Calc. phos. (chronic dosage) helps to balance the metabolism.

Chinese medicine

Job's tears and shiitake mushrooms are recommended: 1 tsp of each food, finely chopped, should be added to a cat's food daily. Beetroot juice (5 ml [1 tsp] daily) may also be helpful.

supplements

The following vitamins will help to strengthen the immune system, and to detoxify the poisons produced by cancerous tissue (the amounts indicated by each are daily doses): Vitamin A (500 iu); B-complex vitamins, as Brewer's yeast (1 tsp); Vitamin C (500 mg); and Vitamin E (50 iu). Garlic, royal jelly, chlorella and aloe vera given by mouth also help to fight cancer.

natural therapies prolong life

Cancer often fails to respond to conventional medicine, although a course of chemotherapy and radiotherapy, or surgery to remove a malignant tumour, may be appropriate in some instances. Natural medicines can be of great help in many cases of tumours in cats, and as a result I am asked to treat a large number of cancer victims. Some of these, sadly, are beyond help, but sometimes a surprising improvement does occur. The effect of the natural medicines may be a complete remission, or, more often – as in Desmond's case – simply giving a better quality of life for longer.

Desmond was a handsome tabby, but he was disfigured by a skin cancer on his face, below the right eye. As the tumour was too widespread to remove or to treat using conventional means, Desmond was referred to me for natural therapy with the prognosis of having only four weeks to live.

I gave him as much of a chance as possible by using a range of natural medicines and supplements. These comprised the Bach flower essences Hornbeam and Crabapple to strengthen and cleanse, homoeopathic Echinacea (chronic dosage) to boost the immune system, injections of Mistletoe extract twice weekly into the tumour, and Vitamins A, C, E and B-complex added to food daily (see opposite for dosage).

For some time, progress was good. Initially the tumour shrank in size by about one-third, and Desmond was bright and breezy. After four weeks the tumour, sadly, began to regrow, but only very slowly. Six months after I first saw him, Desmond was still very well in himself, and eating normally, but with what was by now an extensive tumour. Within a few more weeks the cancer began to ulcerate and become infected, and the decision was taken to bring Desmond's life to an end.

I imagined that his owners would be disappointed that I had not been able to cure the cancer, but instead they were delighted that I had been able to give Desmond – and them – the benefit of those extra six months of good-quality life. This particular case demonstrates very effectively that, although natural medicines may not always have the complete ability to cure, something positive will generally result from their use – and often where treatment with conventional drugs has proved unsuccessful.

parasites

Parasites are creatures that live on or in another animal and feed on it in some way. A healthy lifestyle and a balanced, natural diet should help to ensure that parasites are kept to a minimum, but even the healthiest, fittest cat will occasionally be host to internal parasites such as worms, and to external (surface-dwelling) parasites.

Fleas are especially common, and may not only cause irritation but also pass tapeworms on to cats (see page 117). Natural medicines can play an important role both in preventing parasites, and in resolving any infestation that does occur.

fleas, lice and ticks

These are all surface-dwelling parasites. Fleas are small, dark brown insects that run rapidly through the fur. Lice are tiny, grey insects that move very slowly and are often found in clusters, particularly on the ear flaps. Ticks resemble smooth, grey warts: they fix their mouthparts into the skin and do not move.

Signs and symptoms Visible evidence of parasites; an affected cat may also scratch and groom excessively and, if he or she is hypersensitive to flea bites (ie allergic to flea saliva), there may be raised, red bumps on the skin.

aromatherapy
Cedarwood, Eucalyptus, Terebinth, Lemon, Rosemary, Lavender and Mint all help to prevent external parasites. They can be given by massage or added to water (three drops per 150 ml [¼ pt] water) and combed or brushed into the fur.

homoeopathy
Sulphur: one dose should be given weekly to prevent flea infestations. Pulex (chronic dosage) is a soothing treatment for flea irritation.

herbal medicine
Pennyroyal, Tansy and Fleabane are flea-repelling herbs. The dried or fresh herbs can be sprinkled around the edges of carpets and on the cat's bedding. Garlic is also very effective: ⅓ chopped clove should be added to food daily.

minor therapies
supplements
Brewer's yeast may be given by mouth, or brushed into the fur. Apple-cider vinegar, at a rate of 5 ml (1 tsp) per 600 ml (1 pt) of drinking water is another good preventive measure. A parasite-infested cat may also be bathed in vinegar (⅓ of this to ⅔ water); this will make the coat shine and help to eliminate fleas.

(Opposite) Aromatherapy oils such as Lavender and Rosemary are effective parasite repellents, and make good alternatives to chemical treatments.

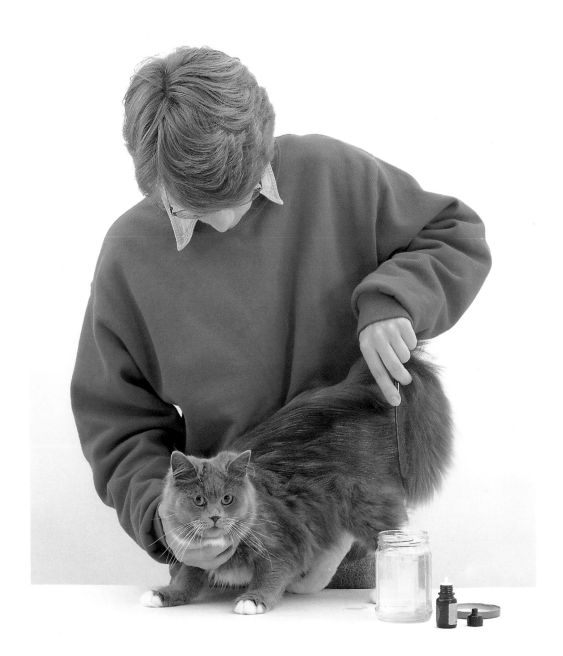

mites

Mites are tiny parasites that can afflict cats in various ways. Two types of mites live on the skin's surface: cheyletiella (rabbit-fur mite), often known as 'walking dandruff'; and harvest mite, an orange creature that affects the feet, legs and stomach areas. These should be treated as for fleas, lice and ticks (see page 114). Two 'burrowing' (mange) mites – notoedres and demodex – can also live in the skin, but are very rare.

The most prevalent mites live in cats' ears. These so-called ear mites can cause intense irritation and lead to conditions such as aural haematoma (see page 67) and otitis media (see page 68), but the following natural medicines will help.

Signs and symptoms Excessive ear-scratching and head-shaking in an attempt to relieve the irritation.

homoeopathy

Sulphur is beneficial for a cat with ear mites who avoids heat; Psorinum for one who seeks heat.

herbal medicine

A mixture of Olive oil and Vitamin E (15 ml [3 tsps] of the oil with 500 iu Vitamin E) should be used to clean the ears twice daily. Rosemary, Thyme, Rue and Teatree may all be given by mouth, or used as a lotion to clean the outer part of the ears. Calendula lotion can also be used to clean the ears; as can a proprietary gel containing Eucalyptus, Thyme, Menthol and other aromatic oils, which kills ear mites.

minor therapies

crystals and gems

Sapphire (liquid remedy) may help.

ringworm

Ringworm (dermatophytosis) is a fungal skin infection that is generally passed on by direct contact between cats.

Signs and symptoms In most cases – but not always – circular patches form in the skin.

aromatherapy

Lavender, Myrrh and Teatree may all be used for massage. Alternatively, any or all of these oils may be diluted with sterile water, at a rate of three drops of oil per 150 ml (¼ pt) water, and then brushed into the cat's fur; this process should ideally be carried out twice weekly.

homoeopathy

Bacillinum, Tellurium, Sepia and Kali arsen. (all in chronic dosage) can help to clear ringworm.

herbal medicine

Goldenseal or Echinacea tincture should be applied to the affected areas once daily.

intestinal worms

Roundworms and tapeworms in the intestinal tract are all too common, especially in kittens. Tapeworms are carried by fleas, so flea-infested cats are most at risk. Other worms found in cats include hookworms and lungworms, but these are rare. **Signs and symptoms** Worms may be visible in the faeces. Roundworms are thin, white, round-bodied and up to 15 cm (6 in) long; tapeworms appear as flat, short segments (the main tapeworm remains in the intestine).

remedies help to control worms

There seemed to be no particular reason why Sage should be so afflicted by worms. She was an ordinary tortoiseshell cat, in good general health, did not go outdoors a great deal, did not eat mice or birds – but she kept on passing roundworms and tapeworms in her faeces. After each conventional worming dose she would be clear for a few days, and then the worms would re-appear.

Sage's owner, rather sceptical about natural medicines, at first thought I was joking when I prescribed 1 tsp daily of equal parts of grated Carrot, ground Pumpkin seeds, Melon pips and powdered Pomegranate rind. I also prescribed homoeopathic Cina and Granatum (twice daily for three days, every four weeks).

Sage now only passes the occasional worm, and intermittent conventional wormers keep them under control. The obvious improvement certainly removed her owner's scepticism.

Such use of natural anti-worming remedies may not be sufficient to remove the need for conventional worming agents completely, as shown above. However, regular administration of natural de-wormers will act as a good preventive method, and will therefore reduce the likelihood of a worm build-up between conventional worming doses.

aromatherapy

Bergamot, Thyme and Marjoram may all be used for massage when a cat has an infestation of worms.

homoeopathy

Cina and Chenopodium are effective for helping to eliminate roundworms; Granatum or Filix mas is suitable for an infestation of tapeworms. In each case, give one dose twice daily for three days, every four weeks, as a preventive measure.

herbal medicine

Rue may be given as infusions; or melon pips, grated Carrot, ground Pumpkin seeds or Pomegranate rind (1 tsp of each) added to food daily.

minor therapies

biochemical tissue salts

Nat. phos. (chronic dosage) is an effective remedy for roundworms and tapeworms.

Chinese medicine

Fresh papaya and coconut are recommended remedies in Chinese medicine: ½ tsp of papaya (chopped) or coconut (grated) should be added to the food daily.

specific infections

All cats are at risk of contracting infectious diseases, although vaccinations and lifestyle can influence the likelihood of infection. Refer to other sections of this book for remedies for the specific symptoms – such as vomiting – produced by common infectious diseases.

feline leukaemia virus

FeLV affects the immune system, causing a range of symptoms including anaemia (see pages 78–9), and kidney and liver damage.

feline infectious enteritis

FIE, also known as panleucopaenia, is a viral infection that results in acute fever, vomiting (see page 97) and severe diarrhoea (see page 101): these symptoms will lead to rapid dehydration and often death.

feline immunodeficiency virus

FIV (feline T-lymphotropic virus, or FTLV) is related to HIV, the human virus linked to AIDS. The virus damages a cat's immune system, and causes a wide range of symptoms.

feline infectious anaemia

FIA is caused by an parasite called haemobartonella, which destroys red blood cells. This causes anaemia (see pages 78–9) and weakness.

feline upper-respiratory-tract disease (cat 'flu)

This is caused by two viruses. Feline viral rhinotracheitis (FVR) causes coughing, sneezing and nasal discharge (see page 72). It can be fatal. Surviving cats often have persistent 'snuffles'. Feline calicivirus (FCV) causes milder flu symptoms, often with mouth ulcers.

feline infectious peritonitis

FIP is a viral infection that can cause two sets of symptoms. The 'wet' form results in a build-up of fluid in the abdomen, with weight loss and weakness; the 'dry' form causes weakness and weight loss, but no fluid build-up. In both cases, the symptoms may worsen and lead to jaundice (most obvious as a 'yellowing' of the whites of the eyes), vomiting (see page 97), diarrhoea (see page 101) and dehydration.

toxoplasmosis

This protozoal infection affects various parts of the body. The many symptoms include weight loss, nasal discharge, coughing (see page 73), diarrhoea (see page 101) and abortion (see page 108). Toxoplasmosis can be transmitted to humans, so great care should be taken by pregnant women when handling cats.

chlamydia

Chlamydia is an organism that causes conjunctivitis (see pages 68–9), eye discharge, and sometimes sneezing and nasal discharge (see page 72). It can cause infertility or abortion (see pages 107 and 108).

The following natural medicines will be beneficial in all cases of specific infections.

aromatherapy
Lemon combined with Sage may be massaged into the skin.

homoeopathy
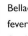
Aconite should be administered at the earliest signs of disease; Belladonna when there is a high fever and the symptoms are severe (both in acute dosage). Specific nosodes to most diseases are also available (for example, Cat 'flu nosode), but should be used only under the direction of a vet. There is evidence that a nosode will help to prevent a particular disease from occurring.

herbal medicine
Goldenseal and Echinacea may both be used as tinctures; ⅓ chopped Garlic clove may be fed daily.

Bach flowers
Rescue Remedy is ideal for any disease whose symptoms have become acute.

minor therapies
biochemical tissue salts
Ferr. phos. (acute dosage) may help.
crystals and gems
Pearl (liquid-gem remedy) may be given by mouth or added to water.
supplements
Vitamin C will help the body to fight specific diseases. At times of acute infection, give 500 mg daily.

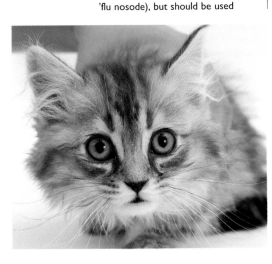

Early symptoms of infectious disease may be mild (such as eye discharge), so regular health-checks are vital.

behaviour

Cats sometimes suffer from behavioural problems, including aggression, anxiety and what is termed 'inappropriate toileting' (spraying urine or depositing faeces in the home, rather than outdoors or in a litter tray). Yet requests for help are not common – perhaps because owners think that a cat's behaviour cannot be changed.

Although cats may not always respond to the simple training methods used on dogs, behavioural therapy involving more subtle techniques of avoiding and controlling unwanted behaviour is often successful. If your cat has developed behavioural problems, seek help as soon as possible – the longer a behavioural abnormality lasts, the more difficult it will be to treat. Your vet will advise you, or may refer you to a pet-behaviour counsellor.

Some behavioural dysfunctions do not respond – or only partially respond – to behaviour therapy, and this is where natural medicines can be very beneficial. Specific behavioural problems and helpful remedies are included in this section.

nervousness

Emotional and mental stress – especially when experienced early in life – can lead to long-term nervousness. Accidents, physical or mental abuse, and even the first vaccination at a veterinary surgery can all lead to anxieties and subsequent nervous behaviour. Some cats are especially frightened of thunderstorms, gunshots and fireworks; some are scared of other cats, vacuum-cleaners or bright lights. One cat I knew was in abject terror of a pop-up toaster. Such anxieties can affect cats at different levels. Some experience a mild nervous reaction to certain stimuli only; others seem to be a little wary and 'highly strung' at all times. Some cats are quite calm and secure as a general rule, but exhibit an almost phobic reaction in specific situations. Events such as a change of home and ownership early in life, or being attacked by another animal, can also spark nervous behaviour. However, some cats do appear to be born with a nervous nature, and it can be hard to change this entirely.

aromatherapy

Regular massage with one or more of the following essential oils will be soothing and calming for an anxious cat: Basil, Camomile, Lavender, Lemon balm, Neroli and Sweet marjoram. If possible, the massage should be carried out twice weekly.

homoeopathy

The following are effective remedies for nervousness (all to be given in chronic dosage): Aconite for nervous problems that seem to begin after a sudden shock or a frightening experience; Argent. nit. for the restless, anxious cat who can be described as 'hurried and worried'; Gelsemium for a cat who becomes almost rigid with fear (this remedy is often given to alleviate stagefright in humans); and Phosphorus, especially for fear of thunderstorms, gunshots and other sudden noises.

herbal medicine

An infusion of Camomile or Oat is soothing (cereals such as oats and barley seem to have a calming effect in many species). Although better known as an ingredient of beer, Hops given as herbal infusions are extremely helpful for a neurotic cat, while Passiflora will pacify and soothe an anxious one. An infusion of Vervain is another good choice for lack of confidence. Finally, Skullcap and Valerian (available as combined proprietary tablets) make a classic herbal calming remedy.

Bach flowers

Aspen is ideal for general background anxiety; Mimulus for fear of specific situations; and Rock rose for severe phobias and panic attacks.

acupuncture

This is a very useful therapy for the nervous cat (unless he or she is too frightened to cope with having the needles inserted!).

minor therapies

biochemical tissue salts
Mag. phos. (chronic dosage) is a very good 'nerve tonic'.

Chinese medicine
Oystershell may be given, as a few fragments crumbled with each meal. Dates and/or longans, given as ½ tsp with food every two to three days, helps to calm a nervous disposition. A few petals of lily flower – known in Chinese medicine as the sorrow-forgetting flower – added to food every few days is helpful for the 'worried' cat.

crystals and gems
Liquid-remedy Pearl is 'nourishing' for the nervous system and will help to calm and soothe a fractious cat.

Bach remedies calm nerves

Bernadette had gone missing. She turned up four weeks later, but kept hiding and refusing food – something had obviously frightened her severely. Giving medication would be difficult but she was drinking, so drops of the Bach remedies Rock rose (for panic) and Mimulus (for fear of specific situations) were added to her water, which was changed frequently.

Within a few days, Bernadette was calming down, and soon eating well and enjoying being stroked. At her next routine check I noticed something strange: Bernadette was a male cat! Remembering that I had neutered her, and that she was definitely a female then, something was amiss. It transpired that the owners had noticed a few changes – an extra white spot here or there – but had put it down to stress. The possibility of mistaken identity had not arisen. No wonder the poor cat had been so nervous, but at least the remedies worked. And, happily, later on the real Bernadette also returned.

aggression

Cats can become aggressive to their owners, to other people (especially visitors) and of course to other cats. A new cat joining a household in which other cats are already resident may be particularly at risk (see the case study on page 23). We all know the sweet, loving cat, lying still while his or her tummy is tickled, who suddenly grabs your wrist and bites it while raking claws down your arm. This type of aggression can be helped by natural medicines.

aromatherapy

Sandalwood and Ylang ylang are both helpful, and may be used for massage or given via a diffuser.

homoeopathy

The following remedies are effective at controlling aggression (all to be given in chronic dosage): Belladonna for anger and biting; Nux vomica for irritability; Staphisagria for feelings of resentment; Lachesis for jealousy; and Hyoscyamus for rage.

herbal medicine

Camomile may be given as an infusion. Skullcap with Valerian can also be administered in this way, or in the form of proprietary tablets.

Bach flowers

Holly is suitable for rage and general aggression; Impatiens for irritability and snappiness; and Willow for anger and resentment.

acupuncture

A course of acupuncture therapy – as is the case with many behavioural problems – can achieve remarkable results in minimizing the aggressive nature of a cat.

minor therapies

T-touch massage

This therapy is very beneficial for aggressive behaviour.

crystals and gems

Pearl or Onyx (liquid-gem remedy) may be helpful: either of these may be given by mouth or added to the cat's drinking water.

Natural remedies can be extremely effective for calming a cat who is acting aggressively towards people or other animals.

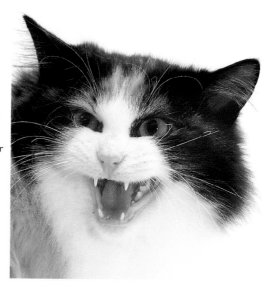

hyperactivity

Certain cats seem to be born with an excess of energy, but a distinction needs to be drawn between normal, enthusiastic high spirits and true hyperactivity, in which persistent wakefulness, repetitive behaviour and manic activity are evident. Stress is probably the most common cause. Hyperactivity can also sometimes be linked to food additives, in which case foods with colourings, flavourings and other additives should be avoided.

aromatherapy

Lavender, Marjoram and Camomile may all be used for massage.

homoeopathy

The following should all be given in chronic dosage: belladonna for an excitable and aggressive cat; Coffea for sleeplessness and hyperactivity at night; and Stramonium, Scutellaria or Tarentula hisp. for a hyperactive cat who exhibits odd behaviour patterns, such as chasing his or her own tail or climbing curtains.

herbal medicine

Skullcap with Valerian (available as combined proprietary tablets) has a calming effect. Lemon balm or Hops may be used as infusions.

Bach flowers

Vervain will calm a hyperactive cat.

acupuncture

This can be very effective.

minor therapies

biochemical tissue salts

Kali phos. (chronic dosage) balances metabolism and reduces energy.

T-touch massage

This has a very soothing effect.

crystals and gems

Sapphire (liquid-gem remedy) may be given by mouth or added to water.

inappropriate toileting

There are many and varied reasons why a cat may choose to distress his or her owner by leaving urine and/or faeces in unwanted places, ranging from dislike of a particular brand of cat litter to fear of a new, bullying cat in the neighbourhood. Stress is the likeliest cause of urine-spraying and middening (defecating in undesirable places) and, in this case, all the natural medicines for nervousness (see pages 120–1) will also help.

homoeopathy

Staphisagria (chronic dosage) is a suitable remedy where resentment – for instance, of a new arrival – seems to be a factor. Ustillago maydis (chronic dosage) may also help with a male cat who continually 'marks' his territory by urine-spraying.

pica

Chewing or eating indigestible material, known as pica, is an activity in which quite a number of cats indulge from time to time. Many kittens enjoy sucking fabrics such as towels and sweaters: this usually stops as they mature, but some cats – especially Siamese – continue this into adulthood. Cats have also been known to eat materials such as cat litter, coal and wallpaper. Any possible physical cause should be investigated, or, if the problem is purely behavioural, a counsellor will help. The following natural medicines will also be beneficial.

aromatherapy
This is used here to treat the fabric, not the cat! Two drops of undiluted Eucalyptus oil should keep a cat away.

homoeopathy
Calc. carb. (chronic dosage) is of benefit in many cases.

herbal medicine
Valerian, given as infusions, should calm an anxious cat with pica.

Bach flowers
Wild rose will be helpful if the pica seems to be the result of boredom; use Chicory if the pica occurs only when the cat is left alone (this is known as 'separation anxiety').

minor therapies
biochemical tissue salts
Calc. phos. (chronic dosage) may help to prevent a cat from eating unnatural substances.

pining and grief

Cats in boarding catteries often seem to feel abandoned, while those moving to new homes may suffer from a form of homesickness. Cats also grieve for absent family members or feline companions, and can even develop physical disease as a result.

aromatherapy
Basil, Bergamot and Orange blossom will help a cat through a period of emotional trauma.

homoeopathy
Ignatia (chronic dosage) – the principal homoeopathic remedy for grief and pining – is invaluable in a stressful situation. Pulsatilla (chronic dosage) is ideal for the shy, reserved cat who has become withdrawn.

herbal medicine
Infusions of Lime blossom will reduce the trauma of bereavement.

Bach flowers
Honeysuckle is helpful for feelings of homesickness and pining; Walnut helps at times of transition in life.

minor therapies
T-touch massage
This is beneficial in many cases.

travel sickness

True motion sickness is probably less common than anxiety and apprehension about travelling. However, many cats suffer from one or both, or from a combination of these two aspects of travel problems. As with many behavioural dysfunctions, prevention is always better than cure where anxiety about travelling is concerned. If you obtain your cat as a kitten, and he or she is apprehensive when travelling by car, try to carry out a programme of acclimatization. Begin by simply placing the kitten in his or her travelling basket in the car for short periods while it is stationary; feeding in the car may also be a good idea. When the kitten is used to this, turn on the engine for a few minutes. Gradually start to make short trips, until the kitten shows no anxiety. The travelling basket should be properly secured – on the back seat with a seat belt, or in a footwell – so that it cannot slide about.

For a cat who does genuinely suffer from motion sickness, finding the solution may be a question of trial and error, as every cat is different and certain remedies may work better than others (hanging bunches of parsley in the car is one odd remedy that has proved successful with some cats!). The following natural remedies in particular are helpful in many cases.

aromatherapy
Sweet fennel, Peppermint and Camomile all have beneficial effects.

homoeopathy
Cocculus, Borax and Petroleum are very effective; Tabacum is particularly good for seasickness and airsickness (all remedies should be given in acute dosage before the journey).

herbal medicine
Peppermint helps to prevent anxiety and apprehension.

Bach flowers
Scleranthus is helpful in many cases.

minor therapies
biochemical tissue salts
Kali phos. (chronic dosage) will help to alleviate nausea.

supplements
B-complex vitamins can be an effective dietary supplement for a cat who is prone to travel sickness. These may be given in the form of Brewer's yeast (¼ tsp daily). Long-term supplementation is beneficial.

appendix

Some homoeopathic remedies are commonly known by abbreviations of their Latin names, and have been included in these abbreviated forms throughout this book. The abbreviations and full names of the remedies used are listed below.

Abbreviation	Full name	Abbreviation	Full name
Acid. nit.	Acidum nitricum	Hydrastis	Hydrastis canadensis
Acid. phos.	Acidum phosphoricum	Ipecac. syrup	Ipecacuanha
Acid. sal.	Acidum salicylicum	Iris vers.	Iris versicolor
Aconite	Aconitum napellus	Kali arsen.	Kali arsenicosum
Ant. crud.	Antimonium crudum	Kali bich.	Kali bichromium
Argent. nit.	Argentum nitricum	Kali carb.	Kali carbonica
Arsen. alb.	Arsenicum album	Kali chlor.	Kali chloricum
Baryta carb.	Baryta carbonica	Kali mur.	Kali muriaticum
Bryonia	Bryonia alba	Kali sulph.	Kali sulphuricum
Cactus grand.	Cactus grandiflorus	Lycopodium	Lycopodium clavatum
Calc. carb.	Calcarea carbonica	Mag. phos.	Magnesia phosphorica
Calc. fluor.	Calcarea fluorica	Merc. cor.	Mercurius corrosivus
Calc. phos.	Calcarea phosphorica	Merc. sol.	Mercurius solubilis
Carduus	Carduus marianus	Nat. mur.	Natrum muriaticum
Caulophyllum	Caulophyllum thalictroides	Pulsatilla	Pulsatilla nigricans
Chelidonium	Chelidonium majus	Plumb. met.	Plumbum metallicum
Cocculus	Cocculus indicus	Rhus tox.	Rhus toxicodendron
Colchicum	Colchicum autumnale	Ruta grav.	Ruta graveolens
Conium mac.	Conium maculatum	Tarentula hisp.	Tarentula hispanica
Cuprum met.	Cuprum metallicum	Thuja	Thuja occidentalis
Echinalea	Echinalea augustifolia	Ver. alb.	Veratrum album
Ferrum met.	Ferrum metallicum	Viscum alb.	Viscum album
Hepar sulph.	Hepar sulphuris calcareum	Zinc. met.	Zincum metallicum

acknowledgements

Reed Illustrated Books would like to thank Jane Burton (and her cats Blossom, Cosmos, Monty and Pansy), Jackie Chambers and Kate Dunning for their help with photography; and Linnea Taylor for her assistance with plant material.

ILLUSTRATIONS: Greg Poole 8–9, 50–1; Annette Whalley 26

PHOTOGRAPHS: Mary Evans Picture Library/John Cutten 21; Reed International Books Ltd/Jane Burton 1, 2–3, 10 bottom right, 11, 17, 18, 19, 23 left, 23 right, 24, 29, 32, 33, 38, 39, 42, 48, 49 centre, 49 top, 49 bottom, 55 left, 55 right, 62, 65 top, 65 bottom, 69 left, 69 bottom, 82, 85, 86, 88, 92, 96, 108, 109, 115; Peter Chadwick (courtesy of Hahnemann Museum) 13; Ray Moller front jacket; Warren Photographic/Jane Burton 119, 122; Kim Taylor 74

index

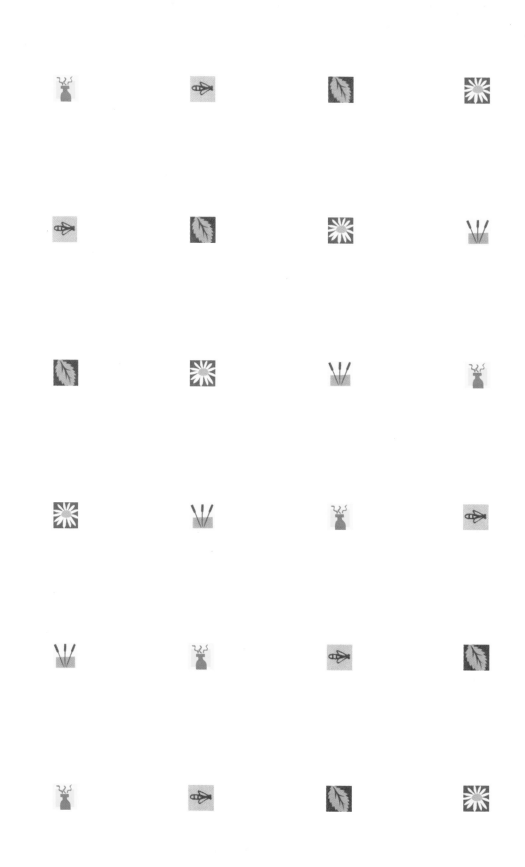